CLEAR IT

MASTER YOUR ENERGY AND TAKE YOUR POWER BACK BY RELEASING WHAT IS ATTACHED TO YOU

BY DR. JAY DAVIDSON

Dr. Jay Davidson

Clear It

Information provided in this book is for educational purposes only and is not intended to replace the recommendations of a qualified healthcare professional. The information in this book does not diagnose, treat, or cure any disease.

DrJayDavidson.com
870 N. Miramar Ave #240
Indiatlantic, FL 32903

Printed in the United States of America

1st Printed Edition

TABLE OF CONTENTS

Table of Contents **5**

Acknowledgments **9**

Foreword **11**

Introduction **12**

The Purpose **17**

Chapter 1. How the Clear It Template Can Help You **19**

Bad Coping Habits and Addictions 19
Being Aware Of Your Symptoms 21
Health Problems 21

Chapter 2. Clear It Template **25**

What Do You Want To Clear? 25
Before Assessment 25
Clear It Template 26
What I Notice From The Clear It Template 30
What Did You Notice? 30

Chapter 3. Everything is Energy **32**

Science Says We Are Empty Space 32
Forms of Energy 36
Helping Others 38
Are There Distance Limitations? 39
What Is The Clear It Template? 40

Chapter 4. Explaining The Clear It Template **41**

Comprehension 41

Part A *42*

Part B *43*

Part D *47*

Part E *49*

Part F *49*

Part G *51*

Part H *62*

Part I *65*

Part J *86*

Part K *87*

Part L *96*

Part M *97*

Part N *98*

Part O *98*

Part P *99*

Part Q *101*

Part R *103*

Part S *104*

Part T *104*

Part U *106*

Part V *110*

Part W *110*

Part X *112*

Part Y *113*

Part Z *115*

Part AA *116*

Part BB *117*

Part CC *118*

Part DD *120*

Chapter 5. When the Clear It Template is Done **122**

Adapting To The Change That Happened 122

Chapter 6. What To Do When Stuck? **124**

The Breakthrough 124

Chapter 7. How To Go Deeper in Your Release **126**

Timeline Your Life 126

Chapter 8. Save Time **129**

What Do the Bolded Words Mean? 129

About the Author **130**

Can I Ask You For a Favor? **131**

References **132**

ACKNOWLEDGMENTS

I am incredibly grateful for all my experiences and the people I have met and interacted with. I am amazed at my private conversations with health practitioners who have had experiences of seeing, feeling, sensing, and dealing with attachments and strange energies related to their patients. I appreciate all the writers and presenters for all the information I have consumed and been exposed to.

I must thank my mom, Bonnie, for planting the seed of the idea of attachments impacting humans in 2017. Erina Cowan, thank you for being patient with all my questions when I heard you speak in early 2019. My good friend Peter Seymour Howe has spent countless hours on the phone with me regarding this topic. My dear friends and fellow health practitioners Dr. Todd Watts and Dr. Nick Ellenson are like brothers to me and crazy enough to hear me verbalize my discoveries along the way and to help shape this book. Thank you to Dr. Todd Watts for also teaching me to use the resonate test, as it has been an incredible tool I use daily. Dr. Jere Rivera-Dugenio, thank you for working to create the BioRegenesis Academy, where he teaches Quantum Morphogenetic Physics.

Lastly and most of all, my wife Heather and daughter Leela. You are both such bright, incredible souls. I am thankful for every moment I spend with both of you!

FOREWORD

The journey of energy clearing is a deep exploration into our core essence, the Source Consciousness Field, which is scalar morphogenetic energy. From my own near-death experience, culminating in developing The RASHA™ technology that has shown the profound impact of unlocking our intron DNA's potential. The "Clear It Template" by Dr. Jay Davidson offers a comprehensive guide to navigating and optimizing our multidimensional energies, resonating with the principles I've experienced. It's a holistic approach to healing, consciousness elevation, and harnessing scalar morphogenetic energy. I endorse this template, trusting it brings you clarity and transformation.

In service to humanity and its untapped potential,

Dr. Jere Rivera-Dugenio, Ph.D.

INTRODUCTION

It was December of 2019 when I was standing 25 feet above the ground on my house roof in Puerto Rico, measuring to see how many solar panels I could fit. I suddenly started seeing spots in my vision as if I had just stared at the sun during the middle of the day. Every direction I turned on the roof looked the same, spots everywhere, and I wondered from my health background if I was getting a detached retina or having a stroke.

I slowly climbed down off the roof and told my wife inside the house that I did not feel well and that I had no idea what was going on. I cannot see; there are blurry spots everywhere I look. I got some distilled water and put some minerals in it to drink in case I was dehydrated. I also thought maybe I was too stressed from work and just needed to sit in our massage chair in our bedroom for a short reset. I laid in the chair to release any tension and stress, hoping my vision would normalize. After a 20-minute session, I had no positive changes and only developed a pounding and piercing headache in what felt like the very middle of my brain.

The progression of symptoms happened so quickly that I did not even have time to process and worry about whether I was going to have to go into the Puerto Rican medical system, which was not known for any stellar service and technology.

I went and laid down on my bed, grabbed my phone, and texted my practitioner friend Peter Seymour Howe. An experienced energy practitioner whom I had met two months prior at our first Exponential Clinical Outcomes (ECO) health practitioner seminar. Below is what I texted

Clear It

Peter…

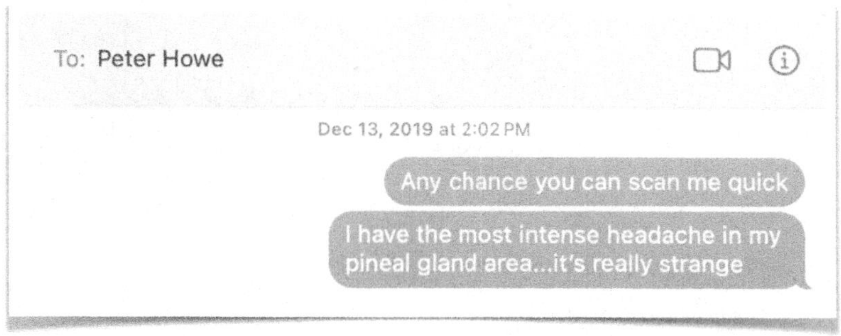

Due to the pain and intensity, I passed out in my bed. I can count on one hand the number of times I have ever napped as an adult during the day; needless to say, I am not a napping type of person. My typical day is jumping out of bed when I wake up and going strong until bedtime.

Twenty-five minutes after texting Peter, my phone right next to me rings and wakes me up. Peter answers as he always does, very happy and energetic. “Hey man! What’s going on with you?!”

As I attempt to explain what I am feeling in my head and that I cannot see, he tells me on the phone that he is picking up that I have attachments on my optic nerve deep in my head. He informed me that it was most likely causing my vision issues and the killer headache. He tells me to give him a minute while he creates space for me to breathe. Within moments, my headache went from a 10 out of 10 on a pain scale to a 4 out of 10. Then he says, "Let’s call Archangel Michael in for some assistance and send these attachments back to the Christ grid.”

As you can see from our follow-up texts, within 2 hours, my pain was already down to a 2 out of 10.

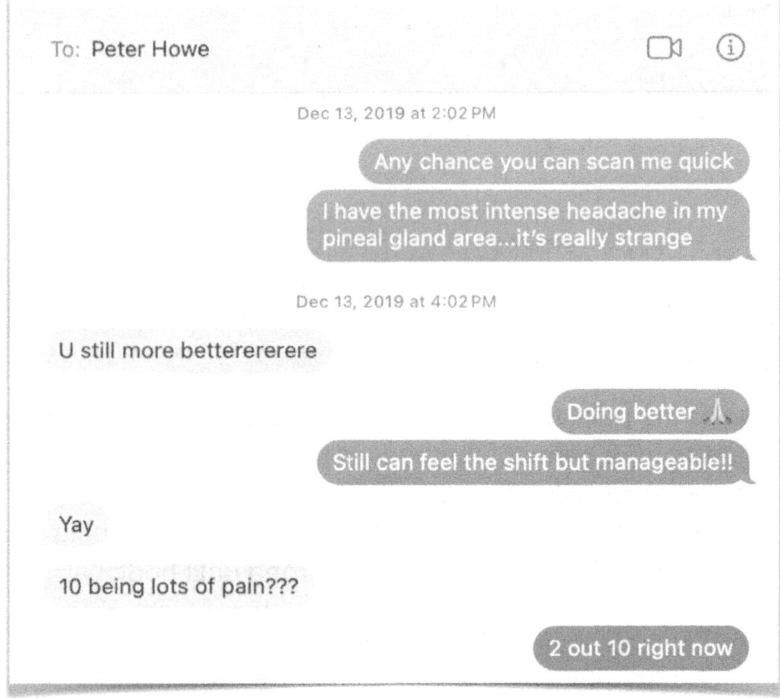

Anatomically speaking, the optic nerve goes from each eye and connects in the middle of the brain at the optic chiasm, not too far from the pineal gland where I initially felt the pain was coming from.

Peter told me my field was wide open with the audience when he saw me on stage presenting at the conference a couple of months ago. He said I must be aware of this as practitioners connected different energies to me. I did not quite get what he was explaining at the time, but later, I would have experiences to shape that explanation better.

After the roof event, I remembered multiple moments in my home office where I would have to double look at the computer monitor as there were spots in my vision's line of sight. My office at the time was a recording studio room with no windows, essentially a dark cave in the lower level of our three-story house so I could maintain focus, no noise, and avoid interruptions.

As with most things in life, those brief moments of spots I had previously experienced in my vision indicated that something was not entirely correct. I did not know what the momentary vision issues were, and it took a crisis-type moment while I was on the roof of my house on a hot Caribbean island and my friend Peter Seymour Howe to connect the dots.

I firmly believe that most of the symptoms we experience are our bodies communicating with us. Your body gives you symptoms that start as a whisper, then progress to a talking level conversation, to then yelling. If you ignore the communication from your body or have not figured out what the body is trying to communicate with you, then a major crisis happens. It is interesting to see how it often takes a crisis-type event for someone to listen to their body's communication and to make changes in their life.

Other practitioners, I have taught the Clear It Template to have stated that this is life-changing information that everyone can benefit from!

I had privately created the Clear It Template for my passion project and then used it for my family and friends. The results and feedback I got seemed too good to be true. I started feeling that because I cracked the code, I had to share it with the world. I worried that with my full-time job in my company, CellCore Biosciences, which I co-founded with Dr. Todd Watts in 2017, that I wouldn't have time to do this project. However, it dawned on me that I was not meant to clear everyone else's baggage, traumas, and energies— I was meant to create the template and teach the methodology through this book so that people could learn to help themselves. Furthermore, this clearing template goes hand-in-hand with my work at CellCore for full-body physical, emotional, and spiritual cleansing.

I believe the responsibility falls on each of us individually to release our own accumulated baggage and traumas. If you do not take the time and energy to do this yourself, you will be limited in how well you get. No one will care more for your health than you do. It is your responsibility. Responsibility is the "ability to respond." How are you going to respond to this? Act and have the transformation you have been looking for.

This book is the resource I would want if I were you. It's time to release the shackles holding you back from being your true self!

THE PURPOSE

This book aims to give you a template you can immediately start using to take your energy back. There are ideas in this book that do not initially come from me. I will do my best to give appropriate credit to all who have had an impact.

I was given the gift of being able to sift through vast amounts of information and put it together into a usable and straightforward framework for learning and implementing. There are many breakthroughs I have figured out along the way, which are included in this book. This is the first book of its kind that I am aware of.

When my wife nearly died after my daughter was born in 2012, the road to recovery was rough. One thing she would repeatedly say that I eventually finally heard was, "Jay, it is always the weird energy stuff that seems to work the best."

I am not here to change or step on your current religious, church, or spiritual beliefs. There are over 4,200 variations of religion and spiritual traditions on earth.[1] You believe what you want to believe. I completely respect those beliefs. This book is a template to consider, use, provoke thoughts, and modify to how you see fit. I come from a Christian upbringing and background, so take that with a grain of salt as you read this book.

When writing this book, I assume there is a creator and that we are not here by the typical scientific secular view. I also believe that there are higher powers that can assist us.

I also want to be clear that I do not believe in asking for

something to come into you at any point. You should also avoid making any deals with any spirits or unseen energies!

Even if you do not agree with everything in this book, take the pieces that fit for you. It is the same thing I do when I consume content.

ENJOY!

Chapter 1. How the Clear It Template Can Help You

Bad Coping Habits and Addictions

If you have a dog, you have probably seen it shake its entire body. If you pay attention, you likely notice patterns of when it shakes. Of course, when it gets wet or it starts to rain, it will usually shake to clear the water off its back.

Sweet Pea, our family dog, part miniature poodle and part chihuahua, will always shake when she wakes up. She will often shake after someone pets her. After she crashes into something or misjudges an athletic jump, she will shake, too. As I have watched and observed her doing this repeatedly, I believe that she is doing this movement to reset her energy and shake anything off that is not hers. Dogs appear to "shake off" stress, tension, etc.

Other animals will do this as well; birds will fly into windows and, if not injured, will get back on their feet, shake their feathers, and fly away.

Although you do not see humans typically shake like animals do, we build habits to either release those feelings and experiences or drive those feelings and experiences deeper into our being in an attempt not to feel them anymore.

When researching how humans can readjust their energy, the most common methods are the following:

- Exercise and stretching
- Spending time in nature
- Breathing exercises

- Getting some sunlight
- Prayer or meditation
- Creative expression, such as art, music, or writing
- Talking through the experience and feelings

Bad coping habits that are common in our society are the following:

- Food addiction, such as eating processed sugary foods
- Drinking alcohol
- Gambling
- Pornography or promiscuous sex
- Electronic device addiction
    - Social media doom scrolling
    - Video game addiction
    - Television addiction (news, shows, or sports)
- Illegal drugs
- Prescription drugs such as opioids
- Reckless driving
- Isolation
- Self-harm

The unfortunate thing with the lousy coping habits above is that they distract us from our body's communication with ourselves. We numb, divert, or drown those feelings away. When you avoid those terrible coping habits, you will begin to hear what your body is trying to communicate to you.

Suppose you have not been able to break a destructive addiction or habit. In that case, this book will give you the tools to clear and release the external energies and hitchhikers that further push you repeatedly into something you do not consciously want to do. But still do it!

Hitchhikers are the unseen beings and spirits that attach to you or your fields.

Being Aware Of Your Symptoms

The next chapter is getting right into the Clear It Template so you can immediately feel a shift and notice a difference. The question is, what type of feeling or thing should you see in this process?

I am discussing this first so that you can adequately assess how you feel now. What body parts do you feel pain in? What areas of your body do you notice tension in? What parts of your body are continually troubling you?

Health Problems

My left knee is a significant barometer for me. I started to dislocate my kneecap at around the age of 10. Every time my kneecap would dislocate, it would snap back into place on its own. It would then swell up, inflame, and take me out for a few weeks. My parents purchased crutches for me as they were sick of renting them after each injury.

I played football, basketball, and baseball, so I played sports year-round. As my knee continued to get injured, the doctors recommended that I stop playing football in eighth grade. They then recommended I stop playing basketball in 10th grade. My knee got so bad that I was walking into my friend's house and dislocated it from a simple 3-inch step into his house.

The only remedy and solution I was given at the time was knee surgery. They made three small incisions to laterally release the outer portion of my kneecap that was pulling it. They also created a six-inch incision to tighten the inner part of my knee to stop it from dislocating. This not only left me with a lot of scar tissue but immobilized my leg for six and half weeks post-surgery. This immobilization made my left leg muscles disappear.

After removing the knee immobilizer, my left quad muscle was the same size as my right calf. That then signed me up for lots of physical therapy in an attempt to rebuild the musculature. After the surgery, my knee did not feel right, and I had a lot of crepitus and grinding with any movement.

This experience made me realize I was interested in health and wanted to work in the health world. I continued to have knee struggles for the next 21 years before one day, I was reading a book from Maureen St. Germain called "Reweaving the Fabric of Your Reality" when I read the sentence:

> "Another way you might pick up discarnate entities is to have surgery with anesthesia."

It struck a chord that rang so hard that I put the book down and started processing the question. What if I have an entity in my knee from my knee surgery? It seemed plausible as the energies typically in a hospital typesetting do not tend to be the best. I remember when my grandpa was in the hospital before he passed, and he was adamant, telling his kids that he just wanted to get out of the hospital.

The realization that a demon could be attached to my knee from the knee surgery I had at age 17 was a big turning point. As soon as I released the demon from my knee, I could immediately bend it without discomfort. It finally felt like my knee was connected back to my body. I finally started to be able to contract the vastus medialis muscle for the first time in 21 years since the surgery. Despite spending years with physical therapy, chiropractic, electrical stimulation, hands-on bodywork, and squatting 325 pounds, only to always end up in the same stuck place of no muscle growth and the same pain and problems.

I remember sitting in the back of a friend's two-door car in college with absolutely no legroom. The car ride, which was about two hours long, was one of the most painful car rides I had experienced. I thought the pain was that I could not move my knee from the bent position and just needed to straighten my leg. Well, it turns out I had some hitchhikers on my knee from my surgery.

While a body part feeling better, such as my knee, is a more noticeable shift. What if you already feel good, and "nothing" seems to be an issue? I will first say that I believe this to be rare. If you think this way, then there is the potential that you have disconnected from feeling your body. A good friend of mine recently passed away from falling off a golf cart and hitting his head on the pavement while intoxicated. He was an alcoholic and drank a lot of red wine. The alcohol poisoning over the years weakened the region of the brainstem that took the trauma from falling off the golf cart. He immediately developed a brain bleed that they were unable to stop and repair.

When I think back to conversations I had with him about how I did not understand how he was able to stay up so late, drink so much, and neglect his physical body and somehow still function the next day. He had told me, "Jay, I learned to stop listening to my body years ago; otherwise, I would feel too much pain." His passing in a tragic accident was not a surprise to me.

While this example was on the extreme end of neglecting his body, tragically, he left his wife and two young children behind. I do believe there is a purpose for us to be able to essentially cut the feeling sensation off an area of the body.

Childbirth is a typical time for a female to disconnect her consciousness from her physical body to stop feeling the extreme pain that childbirth can cause. This is a survival mechanism so humans can do "superhuman" things. The problem can arise when disconnecting from your physical body becomes a chronic habit. For instance, after a traumatic event or experience where you might have disconnected, you must bring your consciousness back into your physical body and be fully connected. Any level of disconnection for an extended period will lead to disease.

CHAPTER 2. CLEAR IT TEMPLATE

WHAT DO YOU WANT TO CLEAR?

What parts of your life need your healing attention?

Are there relationships you want to heal or habits you want to change?

Two blanks at the beginning of the Clear It Template need to be filled in. The first is to decide whether to do a general release for yourself or target a specific challenge. I recommend focusing on a general release the first time you read this.

The second blank is who are you going to ask for help from? I have put some common choices in the parathesis. Pick what you prefer or resonate with.

There are potentially many words or sentences that might not make sense when you first read them. The rest of the book details each section and why certain word choices exist. You will also see many bolded words; this is done to make the Clear It Template faster when you get more familiar with it.

BEFORE ASSESSMENT

It is time to take a moment and assess the following before reading through the Clear It Template to document the changes you have:

How do you feel now?

What body parts do you feel pain in?

What areas of your body do you notice tension in?

What parts of your body are continually troubling you?

How clear are your thoughts right now?

Write your answers down on paper or type them into your phone.

CLEAR IT TEMPLATE

(a) **I am joining with myself right now regarding ______** (general or specific challenge).

(b) **Invoking the assistance of _____** (God, source, creator, Christ, Jesus Christ, angels, guides, etc.)

(c) **Pulsing** an infinite number of stressors in all consciousness and unconsciousness states.

(d) **Connected with all** people, creatures, events (actions), locations (area, organ, system), physical, chemical, mental, emotional, energetic, spiritual, environment, time, antennas, and receivers.

(e) **In all**: the past, the present, the future, this life, all past lives, all probable selves, alternate time spheres, other incarnations, and parallel universes and dimensions.

(f) **To amplify and reveal all** hitchhikers (demons, entities, disincarnates, incarnates), perverse parasitic unhealthy cords, energies, attachments, holograms, fabrications, and beings; manipulations, mutations, distortions, traumas, previous and current unhealthy commitments, contracts, and agreements; body portals, environmental portals, and protective guarding.

(g) **Deleting, transmuting, and removing all**: hitchhikers, perverse parasitic unhealthy cords, energies, attachments, holograms, fabrications, and beings; manipulations, mutations, distortions, traumas, previous and current unhealthy commitments, contracts, and agreements; body portals, environmental portals, and protective guarding.

(h) **In all**: the past, the present, the future, this life, all past lives, all probable selves, alternate time spheres, other incarnations, and parallel universes and dimensions.

(i) **Connected with all** people, creatures, events (actions), locations (area, organ, system), physical, chemical, mental, emotional, energetic, spiritual, environment, time, antennas, and receivers.

(j) **Related to every combination, in the proper order, as many times as needed.**

(k) **Including all**: consciousness and unconsciousness states, ETHUR, SP°, scaylons, scalar points, levels, dimensions, bodies, Eukatharista body, morphogenetic crystal body, mind, morphic fields, BPR, Sha'Ka'Ras, crystal seals, field, field Generator, UM-Shaddh-Eie, DNA, intron DNA, body encoding system, AzurA dish, holograms, sacred geomancies, and light symbol codes.

- (l) **Along with all** active vows, commitments, contracts, and agreements.
- (m) **If any hitchhikers have not completed** their chosen life path, take them to the farthest depths of darkness right now to complete their life path.

(n) **Lock into everything associated**: Chemical, Physical, Environmental, Mental, Emotional, Spiritual.

(o) **Deleting, transmuting, and removing (everything)** from all consciousness and unconsciousness states, ETHUR, SP°, scaylons, scalar points, levels, dimensions, bodies, Eukatharista body, morphogenetic crystal body, mind, morphic fields, BPR, Sha'Ka'Ras, crystal seals, field, field Generator, UM-Shaddh-Eie, DNA, intron DNA, body encoding system, AzurA dish, holograms, sacred geomancies, and light symbol codes.

(p) **Releasing (everything)** all limiting factors, attractors, attachments, identification to these patterns & identities, especially given by others, and protective guarding.

(q) **Collapsing all those energies into the source grid, back into light.**

(r) ***Reversing all ill effects and filling all voids with source love, light, and oscillations.***

(s) **Repeat as many times as needed.**

(t) **Delete, transmute, and remove all mutations, interference, manipulations, and distortions.**

(u) **Delete, transmute, and remove all detrimental external energies and shift my energy to avoid being impacted.**

(v) **Delete, transmute, and remove all energies being extracted and shift my energy not to allow.**

(w) **Delete, transmute, and remove all fulfilled and non-beneficial**: unhealthy commitments, vows, contracts, agreements, and soul agreements.

(x) **Return to when every combination, in the proper order, as many times needed, had no interference, distortions, or manipulations, and bring them forward to now and hold.**

(y) **Restore and anchor both polarities and all four cardinal directions in everything.**

(z) **Shift the time spheres to reflect the changes made right now**, including the past, the present, the future, this life, all past lives, all probable selves, alternate time spheres, other incarnations, and parallel universes and dimensions.

(aa) **"What a great experience, releasing all** hitchhikers, perverse parasitic unhealthy cords, energies, attachments, holograms, fabrications, and beings; manipulations, mutations, distortions, traumas, previous and current unhealthy commitments, contracts, and agreements; body portals, environmental portals, protective guarding, and related energies, all times. **COMPLETED!** (stamped). **Filled with source love, light, and oscillations."**

(bb) **Reset, realign, and optimize energy and energy flow to the clearing and create coherence with the energies around me.**

(cc) **Adjust my Merkaba spin to the most appropriate eternal ratio and spin speed and hold for as long as is beneficial.**

(dd) **Create coherence with X, Y, and Z planes.**

What I Notice From The Clear It Template

What I most commonly noticed during the Clear It Template were my eyes watering and nose dripping. I always seem to need facial tissues while reading through it. Every morning, my eyes feel rinsed with the tears from the release. I notice my eyes look healthier and brighter afterward, too. There are two parts during the Clear It Template that I will generally feel the most: the "reversing all ill effects" part and the very end of the clearing.

Sometimes, I will yawn so strongly that I cannot keep my eyes open. Or I must reach my hands out to my sides and have a giant stretch. I notice that the intensity of the stretch I feel I need to take, the amount of eyes watering and nose running, or the intensity of yawn is a direct reflection of how important and impactful that release was for me.

My body energetics reset faster after reading through the Clear It Template when I take a few moments to stand up and walk around the house or go to the bathroom.

There are times that I feel a sudden urge as if I need to throw up, and inevitably, it is a burp that comes out, and I feel 100% better. If you ever have Peter Seymour Howe work on you, you will hear him burping and belching as energy clears.

What Did You Notice?

Did you feel agitated before finishing it and then peaceful now? Did you have to stretch or stand up for a moment? Did your eyes water or nose run? Did you yawn, burp, or have to use the bathroom?

If there were specific symptoms you were feeling before

reading through the Clear It Template, how do those now feel? Typically, give yourself 10-15 minutes after clearing and releasing everything covered in the Clear It Template to notice the changes in symptoms.

The following are the most common signs that an energy shift happened:

- Yawning
- Burping
- Eyes watering
- Nose running
- Big breath
- Big stretch
- Gas
- The need to urinate after
- The need to take a poop after
- A wave of tiredness (similar to the sleep window feeling)

If you noticed any common signs of an energy shift, your body communicated with you that this was helpful. If you notice the symptoms you were aware of have already been reduced, your body communicates with you that the symptoms you feel have much to do with releasing energy instead of just diet and exercise.

If you did not notice anything, chances are you were hesitant about what the Clear It Template said and why, which is excellent, too. I am initially skeptical of anything in the energy, religious, or spiritual world, as I do not know everyone's intention or meaning behind things they say or do. The rest of this book details the intention behind each part of the Clear It Template.

CHAPTER 3. EVERYTHING IS ENERGY

SCIENCE SAYS WE ARE EMPTY SPACE

Whether humans are filled with energy or empty space, we can influence and shift it. When humans influence this energy or empty space, we can release the shackles that alter us at the microscopic scale, giving us the ability to function optimally.

What is the physical body composed of? When you look at it from a macroscopic scale, our physical body is composed of about 79 organs.[2] Adults typically have 206 to 213 bones, depending on how certain bones fuse or do not fuse.[3] There are over 650 different skeletal muscles in the human body.[4] All those organs are composed of tissues. All those tissues are composed of cells. The most recent estimates reveal that our human body comprises about 30 trillion human cells and 39 trillion bacteria.[5,6]

Each cell contains water and four major families of small organic molecules:

1) Sugars, also known as polysaccharides or carbohydrates.
2) Fatty acids, also known as fats.
3) Amino acids, also referred to as proteins.
4) Nucleotides.[7]

As we look at what sugars are composed of on an elemental level, they are mostly carbon, hydrogen, and oxygen.[8] Fatty acids are carbon, hydrogen, and oxygen; some contain phosphorus, nitrogen, sulfur, and other elements.[9] Amino acids are elementally composed of carbon, hydrogen, oxygen, and nitrogen.[10] Nucleotides are the basic building blocks of nucleic acids. RNA and DNA are polymers made of long chains of nucleotides.[11] Nucleotides comprise carbon, hydrogen, oxygen, nitrogen, and phosphorus.[12] Water, the fifth component of a cell, is hydrogen and oxygen, as you probably know as H_20.

After reading through that and seeing similar elements repeated, it probably does not surprise you that our bodies are 96% carbon, hydrogen, oxygen, and nitrogen.[13] The breakdown of these elements in our bodies is as follows:

- 65% oxygen
- 18% carbon
- 10% hydrogen
- 3% nitrogen

Less than 4% are all the other elements, such as minerals.

As the elements are analyzed on the atomic level, it is classically accepted that they are composed of protons, neutrons, and electrons. The protons and neutrons are in the middle of the element, and the electrons are the portion composing the outer rings of the elements.

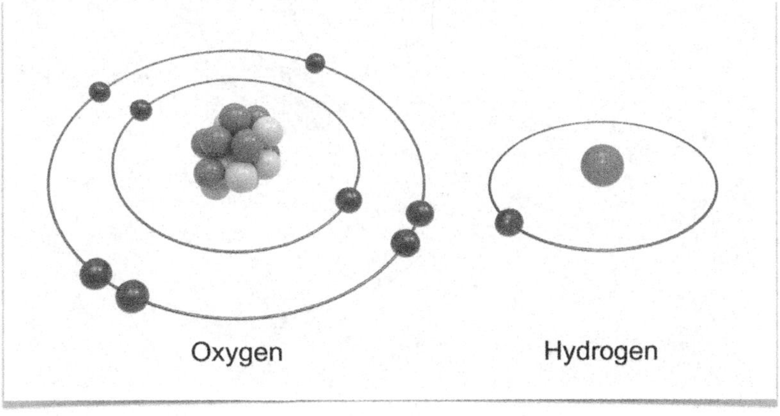

Pictured above are the atomic drawings of oxygen and

hydrogen.[14,15]

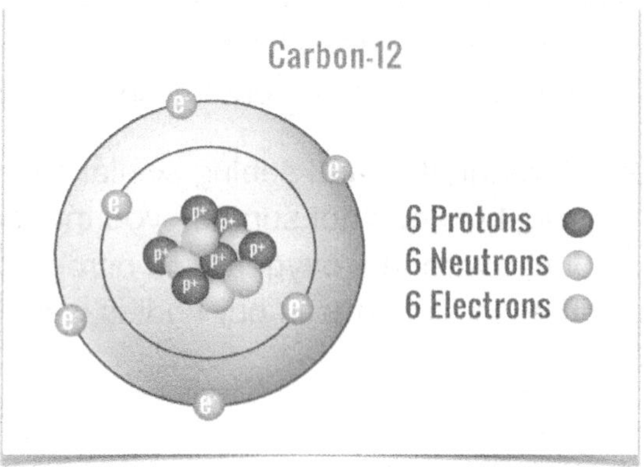

The atomic carbon drawing above is another image showing a different reference style.[16] Atoms are one ångström across in size. Protons and neutrons are 100,000 times smaller than an ångström.

When you Google® "how much of an atom is empty space," Google® tells you that 99.9999999999996% is empty space.[17]

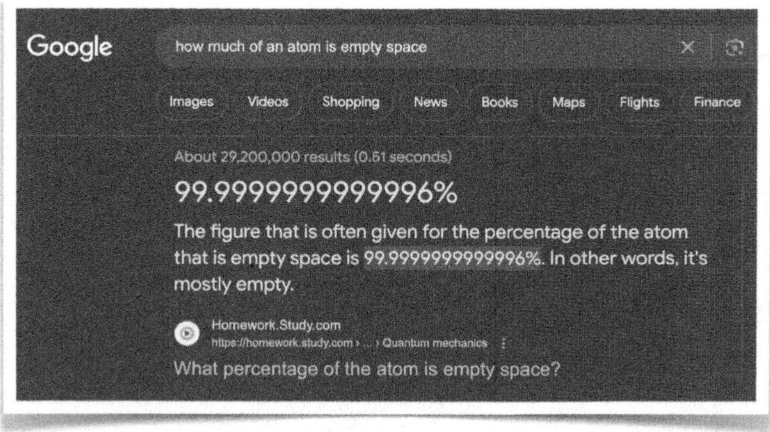

It is strange to think about science saying that our bodies

are mostly "empty space" according to the current classical scientific theories.

I do not believe it is an empty space but an energy we cannot identify with traditional science.

> On a side note, "the orbital model of the atom has not been ultimately proven and, part of the time, must be discarded in atomic thinking. Scientists like Edwin Kaal believe in a structured atom model instead of the standard orbital model. Other scientists believe in more of a dense packing model."[18]

I only bring this up as science is still trying to figure out even what the fundamental element looks like at the atomic level. Anyone who has researched the double-slit experiment and quantum mechanics will know that energy forms can change based on whether someone observes them.

Scientists like Aristotle, Rene Descartes, and Sir Isaac Newton called this energy luminiferous ether. They were also referred to as luminiferous aether or the shorted versions of aether or ether.

In the 19th century, scientists Michelson and Morrey failed to detect the presence of ether and dismissed it. From hearing of these failed experiments, Albert Einstein rejected the notion of the ether. In 1920, while giving a speech at the University of Leiden, Einstein stated, "Recapitulating, we may say that according to the general theory of relativity, space is endowed with physical qualities; in this sense, therefore, there exists an ether. According to the general theory of relativity, space without ether is unthinkable; for in such space there not only would be no propagation of light, but also no possibility of existence for standards of space and time ..."

Four years later, in 1924, Einstein wrote a paper and stated that the "aether of general relativity" is not absolute because matter is influenced by the aether, just as matter influences the structure of the aether. Following the publication of that paper, modern physics stopped supporting the word "aether."[19]

Quantum Morphogenetic Physics refers to this energy as E-TH-UR, aka consciousness.[20]

As stated earlier, whether it is empty space or filled with energy, humans have the ability to influence and shift it. When humans influence this energy or empty space, humans can release the shackles that alter us at the microscopic scale. Humans have the ability to express true health when they release what is altering the structure that dictates the function.

"It always seems impossible until it is done."
~Nelson Mandela

FORMS OF ENERGY

The American Medical Association (AMA) was incorporated in 1897. Four years later, in 1901, the Rockefeller Institute for Medical Research was founded. Simon Flexner was a board member of the Rockefeller Institute for Medical Research. In 1910, Simon's brother, Abraham Flexner, published the Flexner Report, which standardized medical education to petroleum-based pharmaceutical dispensing.[21] This report caused 75% of the U.S. medical schools to close.[22]

Since the last 100 years of dominance that continues today, that dominance is lessening, but it is still there. They state, "The Flexner model remains in place, the foundation of the magnificent edifice that is American medicine."[23]

Thanks to the Rockefeller Institute's influence and belief they created, most normies only believe that a chemical reaction via pharmaceutical pills is what can help with health issues and symptoms.

There are multiple forms of energy outside of the standard chemistry reaction.

Light is a form of electromagnetic energy made up of photons, the fundamental particles of light.

Electrical energy is what charges the human cells. You can receive this energy by putting your feet or any body part directly on the Earth. There is quite a bit of research showing the improvements that happen when Earth donates electrons to your body. There are also electrical devices such as microcurrent therapy, TENS (Transcutaneous Electrical Nerve Stimulation), or direct current stimulation like The Neubie® that can provide electrical energy to the body.

Magnetic energy, which unfortunately has a snake oil-type belief currently cast over it. Magnetic energy is the communication form for our intron DNA. According to the German Nikola Tesla named Konstantin Meyl, intron DNA sends and receives information with magnetic scalar energy pathways.[24] I discuss more about magnets in Part Y of this book.

Scalar energy, also known as ether or E-TH-UR, is the parent of electromagnetic energy. Scalar energy is energy plus information and has no distance limitation. Devices such as The Rasha™ produce scalar energy and other energies, such as sound, that can be used to improve health.

Sound is another energy form with robust health and healing implications. Dr. Jack Kruse says that sound is ultimately converted to light in the cochlea, so light is the highest energy form. Light has great power, but scalar energy is the parent of sound and light and has the most impact. Whether it is sound or sound that is converted to light, healing modalities of sound therapy have made significant shifts in human health.

Devices or machines outside the body can help awaken our body's ability to heal. However, creating a change in your body does not have to require a device or machine. Our brains are powerful scalar energy generators.

> "The human brain is a scalar energy generator that repetitively creates patterns of scalar waves via the activity of thought. According to Nikola Tesla, with two cerebral brain halves (left and right hemispheres), the human being has a scalar energy interferometer between the ears. Since the brain and nervous system processes high-frequency discharges, the human brain can create and detect scalar waves. Thus, a human being can often generate anomalous spatiotemporal effects at a distance and through time."[25]

Energy cannot be created or destroyed. It only changes form. Your intention is powerful.

Helping Others

You can use the Clear It Template on other people, such as your child, your pet, or another person. If it is another person, get permission from them to use the Clear It Template.

ARE THERE DISTANCE LIMITATIONS?

Will it still work when doing the Clear It Template for someone not by you, say 200 miles or even 2,000 miles away? Yes, it will. The Clear It Template accesses scalar energy, which has no distance limitations.

Albert Einstein's famous equation $E=MC^2$, which stands for energy equals mass times the speed of light squared. Nowhere in that equation does it have the letter D for distance. Everything is energy.

Quantum entanglement, which falls within the Quantum Physics portion of science, has been demonstrated with photons, neutrinos, electrons, molecules like buckyballs, and small diamonds.[26] Quantum entanglement is when two groups of energies interact or entangle and will continue to interact at unlimited distances. For instance, if I were to take an electron, entangle it with another electron, and separate those electrons by 3,000 miles away. When one electron alters its movement, the other will simultaneously change its movement. There is no delay, no matter the distance. Quantum entanglement is faster than the speed of light.

The Nobel Prize in Physics in 2022 was awarded to three scientists for their experiments with quantum entanglement.[27]

Tim Griswold, a scientist with a master's in Quantum Physics, has said that once one person is entangled with another person, they now are entangled with everyone that the other person has entangled (interacted) with. For example, the moment that I meet you, the reader, I am now entangled with everyone you have ever interacted with, along with everyone that those people have interacted with. That is what I refer to as quantum entanglement to the next level!

This seems to fall in line with a spiritual belief perspective that we are one and that we are all connected. Also, from a biblical view, we are all brothers and sisters.

How many stories have you heard over the years of the power of prayer for someone who is not right next to another person?

What Is The Clear It Template?

A health practitioner, at the conference in November 2023, where I first taught the Clear It Template to health care practitioners, stood up to share his testimonial about how reading through this template twice completely changed the strength of his heart for the positive.

He continued to say that he cares for all types of people, ethnicities, religious beliefs, and backgrounds. So, depending on the person, the Clear It Template can be a prayer, meditation, energy clearing, or whatever fits in your mind frame.

I have always thought of the Clear It Template as a way to release the past traumas that hold you back from being the genuine person you are meant to be and release the shackles that hold you back that you cannot always see or initially feel.

CHAPTER 4. EXPLAINING THE CLEAR IT TEMPLATE

COMPREHENSION

This chapter explains each sentence of the Clear It Template to give further comprehension of the meaning and intention of all the words. In Chapter 2, the Clear It Template was first introduced, and alongside each paragraph, you will notice letters starting with (a) and continuing to (dd). These letters correspond to each part below in this chapter.

I had an energy testing practitioner say to me once that you do not need to know all the specific details and that research is not necessary when you can simply include all the unknown items and things you have yet to learn when clearing someone.

I disagree with this comment and feel it is an excuse to be lazy. Throughout my clinical experience, including pioneering foundational medicine, many clinicians missed parasites and certain environmental toxins despite being energy testers or muscle testers. As soon as they learned more details about parasites and environmental toxins, they started picking them up, which they previously did not.

Every moment I learn or figure out something new, it takes the clearing to another level. I feel the shift. So, in theory, include what you do not know. However, I have found it most effective as you put in the work and time. The deeper you go, the better results you will achieve.

PART A

(a) **I am joining with myself right now regarding ______** (general or specific challenge).

This first sentence of the Clear It Template is designed to ensure you are clear on your intention. The beginning is who and/or what you are focusing on. The sentence above says, "joining with myself"; however, you can easily change that to joining with my spouse or child. If you are using the Clear It Template on someone besides yourself, I believe it is important to ask that person for permission to read through the Clear It Template for them. It can be exciting to learn tools to make significant shifts in health and want to help the entire world. Not everyone is ready and willing to let go of what they are holding onto and what is holding onto them.

When someone is 20 years ahead of the general world, they are considered crazy. You are a genius when you are two years ahead of the collective thought process. You are smart when you are one month ahead of the general world.

Being in the health field and knowing certain things about health that are not viewed by the general world as helpful. I have learned to keep to myself unless someone asks for help or my opinion. I look at my job as planting seeds, and when that seed is ready to sprout, it is not up to me.

In other words, wanting to change the world and help everyone is noble, but most people will take time for that seed to sprout. And they must want to do it for themselves.

Things are a little different when it is your child, and you have custody of them under the age of 18 (or are responsible).

The second Part A says, "regarding _____ (general or specific challenge)." The blank is to decide whether you will have a general focus or a specific challenge, such as a symptom, like a headache, or a body part, such as a sore hip.

If I focus on a specific challenge, such as my sinuses or left knee, I will read through the entire Clear It Template with that intention. When I am done, I always like to read through it again in its entirety with a general focus on follow-up.

PART B

(b) **Invoking the assistance of _____** (God, source, creator, Christ, Jesus Christ, angels, guides, etc.)

Part B includes the second and last blank to fill in with who you would like to ask for assistance from. I was the most uneasy to present this part the first time I shared the Clear It Template, as people have so many different beliefs.

I am not here to change or step on your current religious, church, or spiritual beliefs. There are over 4,200 variations of religion and belief on Earth.[28]

Although the number of people who follow a religion has decreased in recent decades, **82.8%** of the global population still identifies with one of the world's major religions.

Here's a breakdown of the most popular religions, ranked by their following as a percentage of the world's population:

Rank	Religion	% of World's Population
1	Christian	31.4%
2	Muslim	23.2%
3	Unaffiliated	16.4%
4	Hindu	15.0%
5	Buddhist	7.1%
6	Folk Religions	5.9%
7	Jewish	0.2%
8	Other	0.8%

The figure above shows a general estimate of how the population in the world identifies religiously.[29] According to this, Christianity is the largest religion, accounting for 31.4% of the population. Wikipedia divides Christianity into six main groups.[30] The Center for the Study of Global Christianity says there are more than 200 Christian denominations in the U.S.[31]

To be clear, I did not write the Clear It Template with an atheist or someone who does not believe in a higher power in mind. I created the Clear It Template for myself and decided to write a book to share with those who want to utilize it. Remember, this is a template to consider, use, and modify to how you see fit with your current beliefs.

My belief is that there is a higher power that created everything and is willing to assist us in releasing the baggage we hold. Asking for assistance is different than asking something to come into you or making a deal with something. You hear from people like the Medical Medium, who says that when he was a boy, his dog was drowning in the river and he made a deal with a spirit that should the dog be saved, the Medical Medium would devote his life to this spirit. He calls this the "Spirit of Compassion," which doesn't sit well with me.

My religious background is quite storied, hence my unique perspective on energy and how it relates to religion. I was baptized and confirmed in ninth grade through a Minnesota Lutheran Church, specifically an ELCA. My wife and I were then married in a large Catholic church by a priest in Madison, Wisconsin, who was a dear friend of the family and a priest for the Wisconsin Badgers football team. When my family lived in the Milwaukee, Wisconsin area, I was an elder in a 1,000-person Assemblies of God congregation, the largest Pentecostal denomination. I share this to give you more context about my own journey as it has shaped my beliefs and what this book contains.

(c) **Pulsing** an infinite number of stressors in all consciousness and unconsciousness states.

"Problems surface most under pressure."
~Dr. Jay Davidson

The objective for this part and the related parts is to reveal all the baggage and attachments we have so we can clear them. If they remain hidden, then they stay with us. This part, along with Parts D, E, and F, are associated with the body's stress to reveal its imalances. Part C, "pulsing an infinite number of stressors in all consciousness and unconsciousness states," is designed to bring those hidden attachments and issues to the surface.

Being calm, peaceful, and loving is easy when you have no stress or stressors around you. You can become a completely different person when 10,000 lbs. of stressors are dropped on top of your shoulders. Depending on the situation, other challenges will arise. If someone sits at a computer, they might experience a tightening of muscles in the upper back muscles. If someone sits in a classroom, they might experience a whole different brain chemistry shift non-positively. Every situation is a different experience and stress. Each of those will reveal something that another situation might not have.

By saying that we are "pulsing an infinite number of stressors in all consciousness and unconsciousness states," we are bringing all hidden items to the surface for our bodies to recognize so we can clear them.

What I visualize is starting at the solar plexus area (also known as the celiac plexus as pictured below), as pulsing energy moving out through the body. This also includes the spaces between all the atoms of the body and out through every field of the body. I also push a big breath of air out as I say, "pulsing an infinite number of stressors in all consciousness and unconsciousness states," while visualizing the picture below.

Clear It

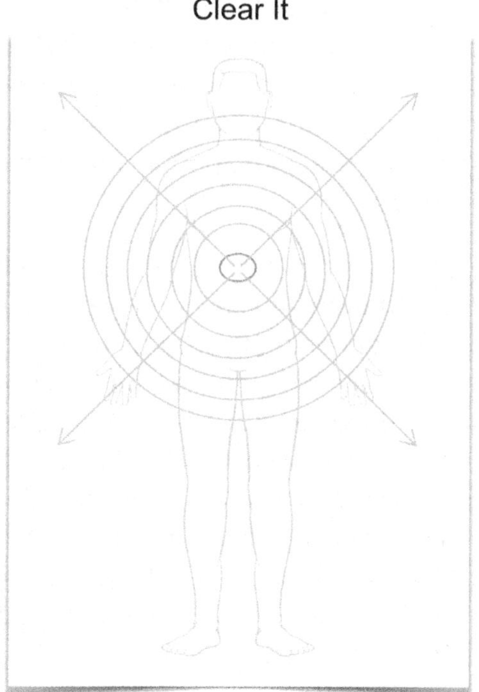

PART D

(d) **Connected with all** people, creatures, events (actions), locations (area, organ, system), physical, chemical, mental, emotional, energetic, spiritual, environment, time, antennas, and receivers.

This part is connected with Parts C, E, and F.

Every event has many things connected to it.

For example, imagine John Doe getting off the phone with his boss, who just told him that he has been unexpectedly promoted to a higher position and will now make double his previous salary. John is ecstatic and decides to go for a joy ride in his car to celebrate. Ten minutes into his drive, his girlfriend calls him and tells him she does not want to be in a relationship with him anymore. At that very moment, a drunk driver crashes into John's car, hitting him so hard he goes unconscious, and an ambulance takes him to the hospital.

Now, this is quite a turn of events that has just happened to John. When you break this event down, you realize many events are happening together, such as getting a raise, breaking up with his girlfriend, being hit by a drunk driver, and going unconscious. The emotions that can be connected to this collective event can be ecstatic, joy, shock, surprise, disbelief, anger, pain, confusion, etc. There are multiple people included in this collective event, from John, his boss, his ex-girlfriend, and the drunk driver, at minimum. We could also include the police, paramedics, and hospital staff.

The goal is to reconnect all those connections to that event to clear the collective event. Let's say someone has headaches that were triggered from a car accident. Despite all the physical body care of a physical therapist or chiropractor, he is still suffering. As all the physical, chemical, mental, emotional, and spiritual connections that are associated with the car accident are revealed, the physical body releases the stored trauma and heals. The collective event and all things associated are the key to fully release and heal.

I have heard instances of people being unable to fully get rid of parasites while doing comprehensive herbal anti-parasitic cleanses until they clear their energetic parasites. Everything is connected. Another thing to note is that anytime one's consciousness leaves his physical body, beings and spirits can enter it more easily. This happens when someone is knocked unconscious or is put under general anesthesia. I am a big fan of only local anesthesia and attempting to avoid whole-body anesthesia when someone is having a surgical procedure. If someone has whole-body anesthesia, I would read this Clear It Template for that person before, during, and after the procedure.

PART E

(e) **In all**: the past, the present, the future, this life, all past lives, all probable selves, alternate time spheres, other incarnations, and parallel universes and dimensions.

This part is connected with Parts C, D, and F.

Part E references all potential times. I have included all the above as "just in case" they exist and need to be included in this release and clearing.

As always, feel free to subtract, add, or modify what I have for words. Timelines are a more commonly referred to term than time spheres. At this moment, I prefer to use the phrase time spheres rather than timelines.

See Part H for a more detailed description of "time."

PART F

(f) **To amplify and reveal all** hitchhikers (demons, entities, disincarnates, incarnates), perverse parasitic unhealthy cords, energies, attachments, holograms, fabrications, and beings; manipulations, mutations, distortions, traumas, previous and current unhealthy commitments, contracts, and agreements; body portals, environmental portals, and protective guarding.

This final revealing part is connected with Parts C, D, and E. One of the most impactful items I have personally and professionally found to cause the most significant positive shift is clearing the energies I refer to as hitchhikers in this book. Hitchhikers include all the unseen energies attached to you, such as demons, entities, disincarnates, and incarnates. See Part G for more information on hitchhikers.

It is also essential to include all "perverse parasitic unhealthy cords, energies, attachments, holograms fabrications and beings." A cord is an energetic tube-like connection from another person or thing to you. You will generally have cords connecting you with all your family members, friends, and those you have interacted with. Many of these cords can be healthy and positive and can remain intact.

It is important to delineate that we want to amplify and reveal all "perverse, parasitic, unhealthy cords." An unhealthy cord can be a source of getting your energy and life force siphoned out of you regularly. For those who want to read more about cords, there is a well-written book called Energy Strands by Denise Linn.

See Part G for more information on "holograms, fabrications, body portals, and environmental portals."

See Part T for more information on "manipulations, mutations, and distortions."

See Parts L and W for more information on "unhealthy commitments, contracts, and agreements."

See Part P for information on "protective guarding."

PART G

(g) **Deleting, transmuting, and removing all**: hitchhikers, perverse parasitic unhealthy cords, energies, attachments, holograms, fabrications, and beings; manipulations, mutations, distortions, traumas, previous and current unhealthy commitments, contracts, and agreements; body portals, environmental portals, and protective guarding.

"Deleting, transmuting, and removing" are the specific words I got from Peter Seymour Howe. Talking to Peter directly, he defines deletion as visually surrounding the energy and disintegrating the frequencies of that energy. Deletion is negating its life force or energetic force. Transmuting is neutralizing it and moving it into light energetics and neutrality. To transmute is to bring something into its light form and unlock all the energetic patterning it holds. It loses its hooks in the form it was in. To remove is to lift the energy up and out and move it back into source light. Transmuting and removing are done in one fluid movement.

Deleting and removing are familiar words and critical in this Clear It Template. According to the Merriam-Webster dictionary, to transmute is to change or alter in form, appearance, or nature, especially to a higher form. Another definition is to subject something, such as an element, to transmutation.[32] Transmutation is to convert one element or nuclide into another, naturally or artificially.[33]

I think of transmuting as taking something harmful or damaging to the body and shifting its energy to neutralize it. If, for some reason, you are not able to delete and remove it from you, the act of neutralizing it into different energy then will not have any impact on you.

The text after "deleting, transmuting, and removing all" is related to things that hold you back from being your true self. Hitchhikers are the unseen beings and spirits that attach to you or your fields. They influence us to do things that we would not usually do. Have you ever done something impulsive and immediately regretted it, thinking to yourself, "That isn't me. Why did I do that?" This situation is likely involving a hitchhiker. I consider demons, entities, disincarnates, and incarnates to be in the category of hitchhikers.

Demons are energy beings without an Earthly incarnation and are purely spiritual.

Entities are organized thought forms.

Disincarnates are human souls that have left the physical body but have not crossed over yet.

Incarnates are human souls currently on the Earthly plane.

The above are my definitions. The lines about how you would classify and define the above can be slightly blurred. Disincarnates and incarnates are sometimes used interchangeably, along with demons and entities.

I do not get caught up too much in the nitty-gritty of the definitions, but want to bring awareness that there are different types of hitchhikers. These can negatively impact your body and your fields, and can also impact you from a distance and in your environment.

A key point is the more you can be aware of, the more you can release and clear from yourself. The more you release and clear, the healthier you are.

It is interesting to hear people's different thoughts about hitchhikers. A friend of my family's who was a life coach for quite a few years told me a couple of years ago that not everyone has hitchhikers on them. The moment she said that, I knew it was the hitchhikers on her manipulating her to say that. The challenge I noticed was that not everyone had the same awareness I had. After my friend said that to me, I knew I still needed to follow my path of discovering more about hitchhikers and how to clear them.

Many religions recognize demons and negative or harmful spirits as well:

- Christianity: demons are considered fallen angels who rebelled against God
- Judaism: in the Hebrew Bible, demons are often associated with idolatry and sin
- Islam: Jinn mentioned in the Quran can be translated as "demons" or "genies" that are capable of harming humans
- Ancient Egyptian: demons were seen as chaotic forces that could harm and disrupt humans
- Zoroastrianism: Ahriman is associated with demons and negative forces
- Hinduism: Asuras are strong beings that oppose gods (the devas)
- Buddhism: some interpretations of Mara depict a demonic figure who tries to prevent people from achieving enlightenment
- Daoism or Taoism: acknowledges spirits and demons, although in a different way than Western demonology

In Daoism, there is a belief that the sanshi or sanchong are demonic creatures or supernatural parasites that enter the person at birth and reside in the three Dantian energy centers. They seek to accelerate the death of their host so they can be freed from the body and become malevolent ghosts.[34]

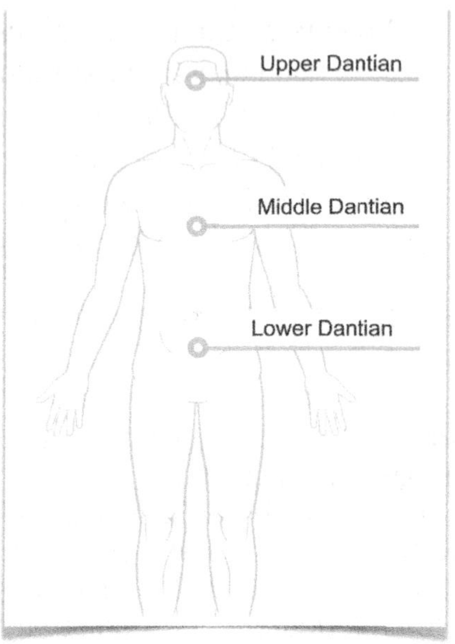

Please note that not all religions view demons and harmful spirits in the same way. I do not claim to be an expert in all religions; as stated before, my background and familiarity are primarily in Christianity. That being said, there are many variations of Christianity too. The Center for the Study of Global Christianity says there are more than 200 Christian denominations in the United States.[31]

It is hard for me to believe that dark, energetic beings attaching to people would be a controversial thought when our culture has them mentioned everywhere. Still, some people think they are just products of our imagination or metaphors for evil.

I like using the term hitchhikers as it tends to have a less polarizing effect than words such as demons, entities, etc. Hitchhikers are referenced in movies such as The Sixth Sense, The Exorcist, Hellraiser, Ghost, The Omen, and Medium. There is a scene in the Trolls Band Together movie in which a troll, John Dory, finds his kidnapped brother Floyd. John Dory tells Floyd, "I'm gonna get you out of here, bro." Floyd responds, "No, you've got to get out of here. You don't understand. Velvet and Veneer are giant, pop-obsessed succubi with no talent, and they've been stealing mine." That part is about 19 minutes into the movie.

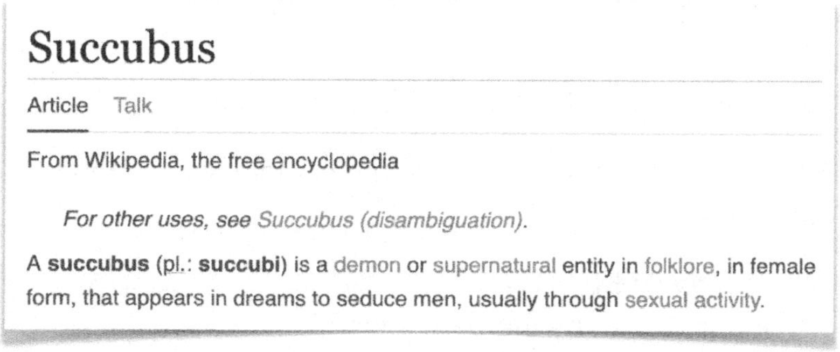

Succubus

Article Talk

From Wikipedia, the free encyclopedia

For other uses, see Succubus (disambiguation).

A **succubus** (pl.: **succubi**) is a demon or supernatural entity in folklore, in female form, that appears in dreams to seduce men, usually through sexual activity.

The image above is a screenshot taken from Wikipedia about succubi.[35]

Television shows that reference hitchhikers include Charmed, American Horror Story, Supernatural, and Ghost Whisper.

The mainstream music industry is riddled with demons, Satan, and darkness. The album cover for Tenacious D's first album, which was released on September 25, 2001, has dark symbology. The front cover features Jack Black and Kyle Gass standing naked, chained to the pole, below the Devil. The position is like what is shown on Devil tarot cards.[36]

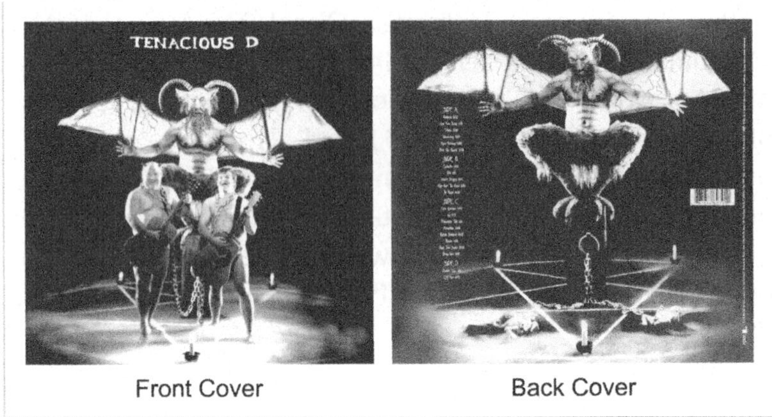

Front Cover Back Cover

Pictured above is Tenacious D's first album.[37]

The following are some songs that contain lyrics about hitchhikers.

Slippin' by DMX

"I'm possessed by the darker side."

Demons by Imagine Dragons

"But with the beast inside, there's nowhere we can hide"

"When you feel my heat, look into my eyes
It's where my demons hide; it's where my demons hide
Don't get too close; it's dark inside
It's where my demons hide; it's where my demons hide"

"Don't wanna let you down, but I am hell-bound."

Inner Demons by Julia Brennan

"Angels don't give up on me today
Cause' the demons they are there; they just keep biting

Cause inner demons just won't go away."

Scars by Tom MacDonald

"They're reminders of the demons who tried their best to defeat me."

Demons by James Morrison

"I got demons I got demons tryna get to me
But they'll never take me down."

Fearless by Goo Goo Dolls

"I'm gonna be fearless, fearless
I'm brave enough to feel this, feel this
I'm running down my demons, demons."

Home by Phillip Phillips

"Settle down, it'll all be clear
Don't pay no mind to the demons
They fill you with fear."

Artists in interviews:

In a 60 Minutes interview with Bob Dylan with Ed Bradley that aired December 6th, 2004. Bob Dylan told the world he sold his soul to the devil for fame.[38,39]

> Ed: "Why do you still do it? Why are you still out here?"
>
> Bob: "Well, it goes back to the destiny thing. I made a bargain with it. You know, a long time ago, and I'm holding up my end."
>
> Ed: "What was your bargain?"
>
> Bob: "To get where, um, I am now."

> Ed: "Should I ask who you made the bargain with?"
>
> Bob: "With, with, with, you know, the chief, uh, chief commander."
>
> Ed: "On this earth?"
>
> Bob: "On this earth and in the world, we can't see."

In an interview on The Oprah Winfrey Show that aired on November 13, 2008, Beyonce talks about her alter ego or possession of Sasha Fierce taking her over.[40,41]

> Oprah: "When does she show up?"
>
> Beyonce: "Usually, when I hear the crowd. When I put on my stilettos, when—like the moment right before when you're nervous and that other thing kind of takes over for you."

The following examples of hitchhikers listed here primarily come from Erina Cowan's Mind Field Repatterning™ course.[42] I believe quite a bit of the information from the course is derived from Raymon Grace.[43] As always, I err on the side of including more in this list than less. Some of these may not exist or be accurate. If they exist and are negatively impactful, I have included them here.

Hitchhiker list:
Black spirals, vampires, beast, henchmen, black witch, witches, warlocks, tengu spirits, poltergeist, greys, Grey imposters, Nordics, Tulpa, Egregore, Negative ETs, space aliens that call themselves gods, Spirit of Death, Negative Spirit Guides, False gods, false light being, potential killer, murderer, dangerous, suicidal, dishonest abuser/alcoholic, weak entity/drug use, negative elemental, machine/artificial

intelligence, primal animal/sex motivated, negative energy agent, predatory STS/lizard brain, reanimated human, controlled victim/food source STS, Controlled STS/food source, NWO clone, NWO zombie, NWO physical, M.I.B., ET clone, negative Draco, Draco shapeshifter, Earth and Geopathic entities, Satan and his 12 Apostates, Baal, and Baphomet.

If you get irritated from the thought of or reading any of these above, there is a good chance one or multiple of these negatively impact you. As you read through more details and greater depths of this book. Going back through the Clear It Template in Chapter 2 is a good idea to release more baggage. Remember, yawning, burping, or having to stretch is another indicator that there is something there or a shift happened.

My definition of an entity is an organized thought-form. The negative thought forms are the ones to focus on with the Clear It Template. Unfortunately, there are many people associated with the dark spiritual arts, and their rituals create many negative beings. My goal is not to be impacted by them. Remember, the more you can be aware of, the more you can release and clear from yourself. The more you release and clear, the healthier you are.

Deleting, transmuting, and removing all: hitchhikers, perverse parasitic unhealthy cords, energies, attachments, holograms, fabrications, and beings; manipulations, mutations, distortions, traumas, previous and current unhealthy commitments, contracts, and agreements; body portals, environmental portals, and protective guarding.

“Holograms” are generally considered three-dimensional image projections created by recording and then reconstructing the light scattered from an object. I am not referring to this when I reference holograms. There was a book published in 1991 by Michael Talbot called "The Holographic Universe." The author suggests that the universe, rather than being composed of solid matter and energy fields as we perceive it to be, could be an illusion projected from a higher-dimensional reality. This holographic projection creates the perception of a solid, three-dimensional world. I am referring to that concept when I use the word hologram.

Even military intelligence refers to the universe as a gigantic hologram. In the now declassified "Analysis and Assessment of Gateway Process," originally written on June 9, 1983, the document states:

> *"The universe is composed of interacting energy fields, some at rest and some in motion. It is, in and of itself, one gigantic hologram of unbelievable complexity."* [44]

This document comes at a time when the military was researching the psychic abilities of the human mind during the Cold War.

Elon Musk has said, "We're most likely in a simulation."[45] I believe he is referring to simulation as an illusion projected from a higher-dimensional reality.

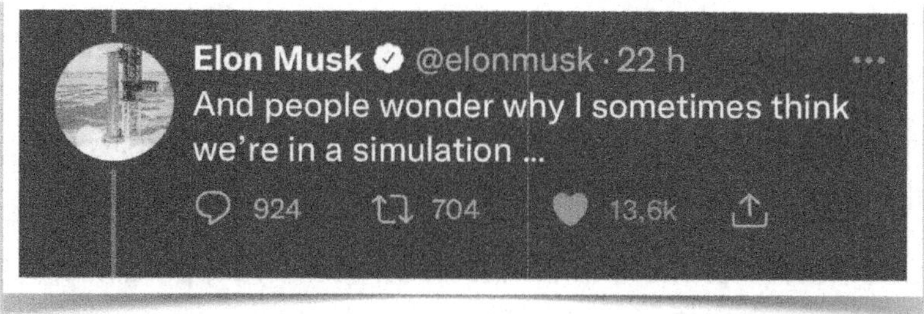

The above image is from Elon Musk replying to a tweet on March 10, 2022.[46] This can be referred to as the simulation hypothesis, often credited to a 2003 paper written by a University of Oxford philosopher, Nick Bostrum.[47]

The video game Pong, released by Atari in 1972, is essentially two rectangles that bounce a dot back and forth. Fast forward to today, more than fifty years later, and we have photo-realistic games and virtual reality technology that people play that becomes more advanced every year. It is not too far off to think that eventually technology will become indistinguishable from reality. If a video game technology becomes indistinguishable from reality, how would we know if we are in a video game or in real life?

The above paragraph is the argument Elon Musk essentially made at the Code Conference in 2016 when asked if we are living in a simulation.[48]

With all that having been said, in case we live in a single hologram, multiple holograms or an aspect of a hologram, I want to make sure the Clear It Template covers any of these circumstances.

“Fabrications” refer to anything that is made up, especially for the purpose of deception.

"Body portals" refer to energetic openings within the body or fields of the body.

"Environmental portals" refer to energetic openings within the environment outside your body or fields of the body.

See Part F for more information on "perverse, parasitic, unhealthy cords."

See Part T for more information on "manipulations, mutations, and distortions."

See Parts L and W for more information on "unhealthy commitments, contracts, and agreements."

See Part P for information on "protective guarding."

PART H

(h) **In all**: the past, the present, the future, this life, all past lives, all probable selves, alternate time spheres, other incarnations, and parallel universes and dimensions.

Part E has the same wording as Part H. Part E references the stressor portion to bring out awareness of the challenges. Part H is the actual inclusion of all "times" to include in the clearing to release.

Time is a multifaceted concept with philosophical, scientific, and personal views. Time seems to have quite the parameters we have put on it as a culture. Some questions to consider are: Is time travel possible? Does time have a flow direction? How does time relate to consciousness?

Clif High has an interesting theory of continuous creation

and destruction model: the universe creates and destroys everything 22 trillion times per second.[49,50] That seems a little wild for me to consider. However, I would not completely rule that out. I think of "time" as a gateway connected with everything. This means that when you impact the now, you alter everything time is linked to, which includes the past, future, and other realms related to time.

Most people are comfortable with future time, the present (now), and past time. As with any section, being told how something "is" earlier in life constrains our mental possibilities. With this programming, it is often easier to dismiss something as impossible or inaccurate than to ask questions such as, "Where does this emotion I suddenly have come from?" and "Why am I so sure of such a stance I have?"

It takes an emotionally mature person to evaluate a question from both sides, even if you are sure one side is right.

I do not profess to have all the truths or claim the responsibility or authority to conclude for you. I have simply included "all probable selves, alternate time spheres, other incarnations, and parallel universes and dimensions" in the Clear It Template in case they exist and in case they are impactful to include in the release. The more range and details the Clear It Template has, the more possibility there will be to fully let go of what is holding us back.

Dr. Jere Rivera-Dugenio, founder of BioRegenesis Academy and a quantum morphogenetic physicist, states that each person has 12 probable selves. Dr. Jere has also indicated that he views possible time as being more time spheres than timelines. That was the first time I had even heard the words time spheres. If time spheres do not feel right for you, you can always replace that word with the timeline.[51]

Reincarnation is the belief that a person's consciousness or soul can be reborn into a new physical body and can be a polarizing word in the religious sense. Certain religions, such as Buddhism and Hinduism, believe in reincarnation. Many Buddhists believe in reincarnation as part of the cycle of dependent origination, and rebirth is seen as a continuation of the karmic cycle. Reincarnation is a central theme to Hinduism, forming part of the cycle of samsara, where karma (actions) determine your next life. My interpretation of Hindus is that rebirth is not just a human form but can be other forms based on your karmic merit. The concept of reincarnation also seems to be popular among New Age-type beliefs.

Most Christian denominations reject the possibility of reincarnation and emphasize salvation through Jesus Christ and eternal life in heaven or hell after death. Islam also does not subscribe to reincarnation. Muslims believe in a single earthly life followed by judgment and an eternal afterlife in heaven or hell based on one's deeds.

I included the words "other incarnations" in the Clear It Template in case this is not my first rodeo for my soul being in a physical body.

The phrase "Parallel universes and dimensions" from the template makes me think about a movie I saw with my daughter and some friends called Spider-Man: Into the Spider-Verse that came out in 2018. It is an animated movie about a teenager who becomes Spider-Man in his universe. He then encounters several other Spider-People from different dimensions. The sequel, Spider-Man: Across the Spider-Verse, released in 2023, also prominently features parallel universes and dimensions as core elements of the movie's storyline.

In case there are parallel universes or dimensions, I again have included them in the Clear It Template. As always, feel free to subtract, add, or modify as you see fit.

PART I

(i) **Connected with all** people, creatures, events (actions), locations (area, organ, system), physical, chemical, mental, emotional, energetic, spiritual, environment, time, antennas, and receivers.

Part D's wording is the same and details how many things can be connected with one single event.

When something traumatic happens, it is easy to forget the other things that are connected. It is human nature to focus on the most noticeable thing. I have found that releasing past traumas is easier and more profound when you link them to minor details and connections.

“People” are referencing anyone else who is or was associated with the thing you are focusing on. I originally had pets and then changed it to animals and finally to “creatures” to include anything that is not a person that might be connected.

“Events” I define as something that occurs or happens.

“Locations” refer to any “area, organ, or system” of the body or field. I included this wording as many systems seem to exist on and around the body that the mainstream has not identified or recognized. For instance, known systems include the endocrine (hormone), nervous, digestive, cardiovascular, circulatory, lymphatic, and detoxification systems.

“Systems” that I have found to exist and have significance include the body development system, the body encoding system (located at the solar plexus), the time encoding system, the social development system, and the projection system, which is related to our holographic reality, the connection system, and the purpose guidance system.

“Areas” can be on and off the physical body from a few inches to 1 ½, 3, 6, 10, 12, or 18 feet. For instance, one of the furthest location areas I have detected related to our body are 12 different receptors that are 18 feet away from the pineal gland at different angles and orientations.

“Organs” includes the two images below, plus more:

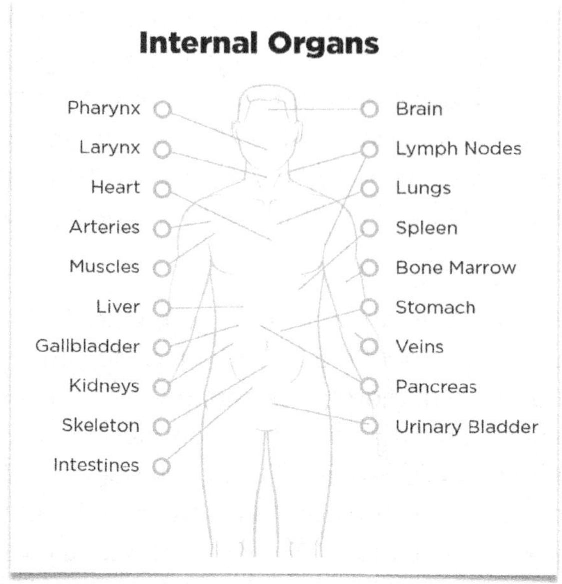

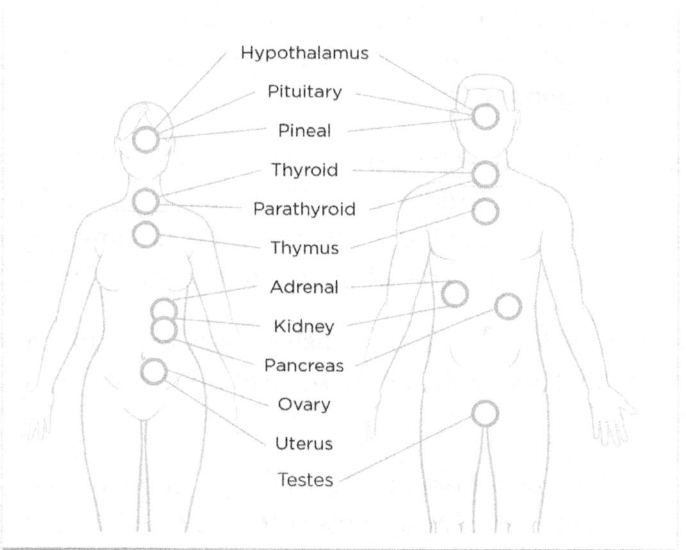

An extremely important organ not shown in the images above to include in your clearing is the connective tissue. The connective tissue, also known as the fascia or the extracellular matrix (ECM), is a vital organ. I believe it is the true "terrain" of the body, rather than the digestive tract. The ECM is the original organ and system of the body that forms first. A paper published in 2021 has a great scientific description of the role the ECM plays in holding the entire body together, along with its impact on reversing aging and cancer.

> "The ECM is a non-cellular component of tissues providing a scaffold for cellular adhesion and triggering numerous mechanotransduction pathways involved in morphogenesis and homeostasis. An increasing number of studies in vivo and in vitro show that changing the mechanical properties of the ECM by re-implanting tissues or changing the stiffness of the adherent substrate is sufficient to reverse aging, accelerate developmental processes, or modulate tumor malignancy."[52]

Even if you have neglected your ECM or it is not healthy, it is not too late. According to Dr. Thomas Rau, the ECM can regenerate in six months.[53] The body has an amazing ability to heal at any age when you remove interference.

It is common to hear about drinking more water to improve your health. Research shows we lose body water as we age.

> "Body water decreases with age, and increases or decreases of body water are common in diseases common in old age."[54]

What is not well known is that the water you drink is not really the same water inside your cells. The mitochondria are the body's primary water generation system for intracellular water, and the ECM is the primary hydration system. There is an important link between our mitochondria and ECM, as shown below with the following excerpts from two peer-reviewed journal articles:

> "Age-related declines in skeletal muscle regenerative capacity have been attributed to the changes in the extracellular matrix (ECM) composition. Therefore, mitochondrial deterioration in the muscle may be implicated in the sarcopenic process, and a possible link between ECM remodeling and mitochondrial dysfunction may be suggested."[55]

> "In migrating cancer cells, ECM composition and stiffness are drivers for metabolic shifts toward enhanced mitochondrial bioenergetics and local mitochondrial accumulation in the leading edge lamellipodia."[56]

New research in the past few years has shown the ECM is the richest sensory organ in the body, with 250 million nerve endings. The skin contains 200 million nerve endings, and the eyes contain 126 million. The ECM is how we feel our inner environment.[57]

"Physical" has a lot of overlap with locations and there is not a clear line between the two. I put injuries, congenital issues, cellular function and communication, non-beneficial memory in water and elements, birth location, and memories erased in this category as things that are not commonly thought about. I would, of course, include anything related to the human physical body itself, such as the muscular or skeletal system, etc.

You may be wondering what "non-beneficial memory in water and elements" means. Research published by the late Luc Montagnier in 2015 showed that water can store and transmit information. The researchers took the DNA of Borrelia (Lyme bacteria) and HIV and placed it into ultra-pure water. They then diluted the sample continuously, like the homeopathic process, until no DNA was detected in the water. They then recorded the water and sent that digital file via the Internet to another lab. After the lab received the digital file, they played the sound file to some new ultra-pure water for an hour. They then put nucleotides into the water and an enzyme called polymerase to catalyze the reaction, which are the ingredients of DNA. They then used PCR to amplify the information and found that they were able to reconstruct the DNA that was 98% identical to the original. These experiments prove that DNA emits Electromagnetic Signals (EMS), that water can store and transmit information, and also validates the homeopathic process, which the mainstream has attacked for years.[58]

Now, with that being said, yes, this is some groundbreaking and fascinating research. However, I will always hold skepticism concerning Luc Montagnier as he made the discovery that HIV is the causative agent of AIDS. The fraud within the "virology" field and the lies and fabrication about HIV back in 1983 are something I will not forget. Now, in all fairness, later in Luc Montagnier's life, he questioned the role of HIV in AIDS.

If you are interested in researching the HIV and AIDS topic uncensored, I would recommend the following books:

- Inventing the AIDS Virus by Peter Duesberg and the foreword written by the inventor of the PCR machine, Kary Mullis
- AIDS Inc.: Scandal of the Century by Jon Rappoport
- The Real Anthony Fauci by Robert F. Kennedy Jr.

For the word “Chemical,” I think about pathogens and poisons we are exposed to through the water, air, food, and injections. Pathogens include pathogenic bacteria, fungi, and parasites. Parasites include nematodes (roundworms), cestodes, trematodes, protozoa, sporozoans, and rope worms. Nematodes and cestodes are always priorities to address first when detected.

Parasites can be found in water and all types of food, such as fruits, vegetables, and meat. This is why it is important to perform periodic parasite cleanses to prevent parasite overgrowth in the body.

Eating bug protein powder or using bug flour is not recommended despite its increased popularity in the last decade. Research published in 2019 examined 300 insect farms and detected parasites in 244 of them. The experimental material comprised samples of live insects from 300 household farms and pet stores, including 75 mealworm farms, 75 house cricket farms, 75 Madagascar hissing cockroach farms, and 75 migrating locust farms. Parasites were detected in 244 (81.33%) out of 300 (100%) examined insect farms.[59]

Poisons can be man-made, such as environmental, like herbicides, pesticides, and fungicides.

Airplanes emit these toxins into the sky and we breathe

them in. On April 17, 2020, the State Agency Official State Gazette of Spain published a State Official Newsletter that announced order SND / 351/2020, which the Spanish Ministry of Health authorized.

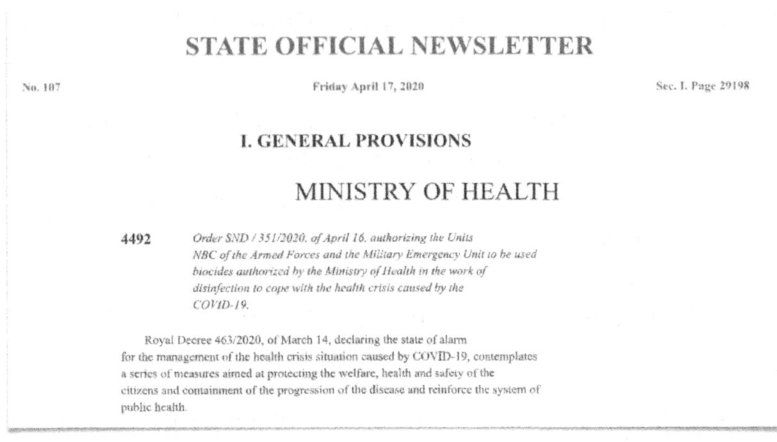

STATE OFFICIAL NEWSLETTER

No. 107 | Friday April 17, 2020 | Sec. I. Page 29198

I. GENERAL PROVISIONS

MINISTRY OF HEALTH

4492 *Order SND / 351/2020, of April 16, authorizing the Units NBC of the Armed Forces and the Military Emergency Unit to be used biocides authorized by the Ministry of Health in the work of disinfection to cope with the health crisis caused by the COVID-19.*

Royal Decree 463/2020, of March 14, declaring the state of alarm for the management of the health crisis situation caused by COVID-19, contemplates a series of measures aimed at protecting the welfare, health and safety of the citizens and containment of the progression of the disease and reinforce the system of public health.

> "Order SND / 351/2020, of April 16, authorizing the Units NBC of the Armed Forces and the Military Emergency Units to be used biocides authorized by the Ministry of Health in the work of disinfection to cope with the health crisis caused by the C***D-19."[60,61]

The key word in the order is "biocide" they are putting in the aerial spray. According to Google®, a biocide is:[62]

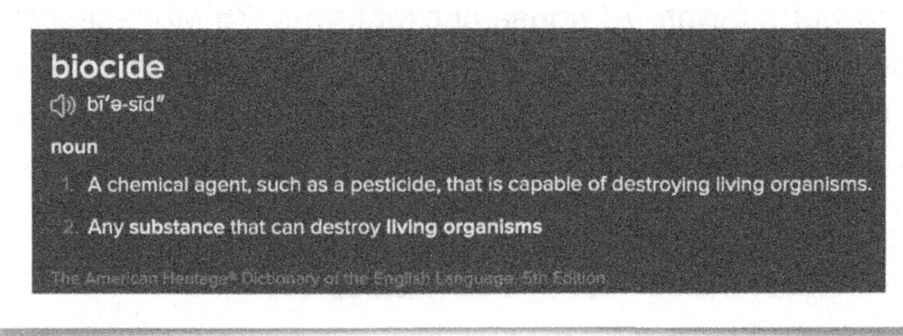

biocide

bī'ə-sīd"

noun

1. A chemical agent, such as a pesticide, that is capable of destroying living organisms.
2. Any substance that can destroy **living organisms**

The American Heritage® Dictionary of the English Language, 5th Edition

Further down in the document, it says the following:

> The NBC defense units of the Armed Forces and the Military Unit of Emergencies (UME) have personal means, materials, procedures and the sufficient training to carry out aerial disinfection, since they are operations that they carry out regularly, with the exception that instead of using Biocide products do it with other decontaminating chemicals. It is therefore

> "Operations that they carry out regularly, with the exception that instead of using Biocide products do it with other decontaminating chemicals."

The government has been putting chemicals and pathogens in the air since at least the 1950s.

> "During the 1950s and 1960s, the U.S. Army conducted atmospheric dispersion tests in many American cities using fluorescent particles of zinc cadmium sulfide (ZnCdS) to develop and verify meteorological models to estimate the dispersal of aerosols."[63]

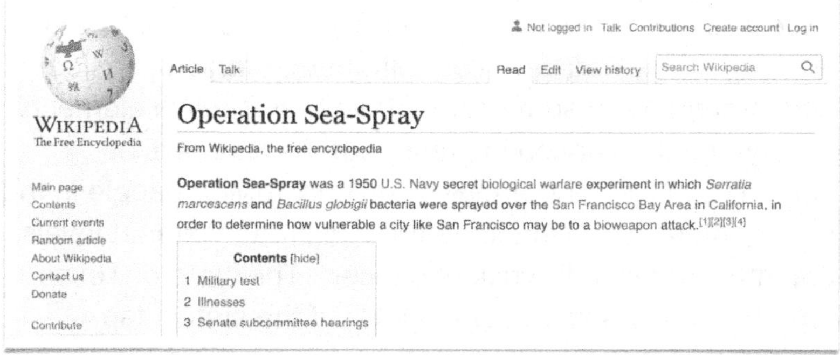

Not logged in Talk Contributions Create account Log in

Article Talk Read Edit View history Search Wikipedia

WIKIPEDIA
The Free Encyclopedia

Main page
Contents
Current events
Random article
About Wikipedia
Contact us
Donate

Contribute

Operation Sea-Spray

From Wikipedia, the free encyclopedia

Operation Sea-Spray was a 1950 U.S. Navy secret biological warfare experiment in which *Serratia marcescens* and *Bacillus globigii* bacteria were sprayed over the San Francisco Bay Area in California, in order to determine how vulnerable a city like San Francisco may be to a bioweapon attack.[1][2][3][4]

Contents [hide]

1 Military test
2 Illnesses
3 Senate subcommittee hearings

According to Wikipedia, "Operation Sea-Spray was a 1950 U.S. Navy secret biological warfare experiment in which *Serratia marcescens* and *Bacillus globigii* bacteria were sprayed over the San Francisco Bay Area in California, to determine how vulnerable a city like San Francisco may be to a bioweapon attack."[64]

The following are things worth researching on this topic of different operations or projects that have occurred in the past.[65]

- 1950: Operation Sea Spray
- 1952-1953: Operation Dew
- 1957-1958: OPERATION LAC (Large Area Coverage)
- 1960s: Project SHAD
- 1961: Project West Ford
- 1962: Operation Fishbowl
- 1950s-1970s: Project MK NAOMI

There is much more to discuss on the chemicals being put in the atmosphere for us to breathe in, but this is different from the purpose of this book.

Other toxins include radioactive elements, which are more harmful than toxic heavy metals. The most significant exposure I find clinically is through the water supply and drinking them. Radium, radon, thorium, uranium, cesium, and strontium are some examples of radioactive elements. Radium contamination in public water systems is at epidemic levels. One hundred seventy million people in the U.S. drink radioactive elements in their tap water at levels that may increase the risk of cancer. The state of Texas reported detectable radium in 80% of the state's tap water.[66]

When Glyphosate is sprayed on plants their concentration of uranium increases by up to 17 times.[67]

Biological toxins are poisonous substances produced by a living organism, such as mycotoxins, which are the toxins that mold organisms produce. Plants, animals, and microorganisms can produce biological toxins.

The EPA (United States Environmental Protection Agency) has a Toxic Substances Control Act Chemical Substance Inventory (TSCA Inventory), which is a list of all man-made chemicals registered by the EPA in the United States. The most recent update as of August 2023 states that there are 86,718 chemicals, of which 42,242 are active, meaning they are still being produced and used.[68]

Many chemicals, such as Agent Orange, are no longer being produced but persist in the environment for years after. Agent Orange is a mixture of two herbicides, 2,4-D and 2,4,5-T, and its production officially ended in the mid-1970s. Dioxin, a contaminant within Agent Orange, can remain in the sediments and soil for decades, even centuries, continuing to cause harm to those who are exposed.[69,70,71]

Certain poisons (toxins) are considered persistent organic pollutants (POPs) and are of particular concern because of their persistence and toxicity. Some of the most well-known POPs include organochlorine pesticides, polychlorinated biphenyls (PCBs), polybrominated diphenyl ethers (PBDEs), perfluorooctanoic acid (PFOA) and perfluorooctanesulfonic acid (PFOS).

An Australian study published in 2022 found that a single five-centimeter (cm) scratch to a Teflon pan, perhaps from a spatula or spoon, released up to 2.3 million microplastic particles.[72]

German researchers found in a study published in the journal PLoS One that nearly 25,000 chemicals were found in one single water bottle.[73,74]

"Mental" and "Emotional" are often used together and interchangeably. I think of mental as a broader scope describing all cognitive and psychological processes, while emotional references more feelings and moods.

"Mental" includes, but is not limited to, attention, analysis, language, logic, memory, problem-solving, reasoning, and thinking.

"Emotional" refers primarily to affective states, feelings, and moods. I recommend reading the book The Emotion Code by Dr. Bradley Nelson for a more in-depth discussion on the emotion category. His technique with magnets is interesting to release emotion, but does not connect all the other pieces tied to the emotions. Dr. Nelson and his wife discovered the heart wall. The heart wall is an energetic wall a person creates around his heart using the stored traumas and trapped emotions to in order to protect himself. This a reason people can feel disconnected from others and the world. Different practitioners have told me that he does not teach the hidden heart wall anymore, which he discusses in his book. A hidden heart wall is another layer on the original heart wall that the subconscious mind is trying to hide from your awareness. I still included the hidden heart wall in the list below, as I would rather include more than less, just in case. He also teaches Body Code™ and his newer Belief Code®.[75]

Items included in the mental and emotional category include the following: non-beneficial conscious and unconscious beliefs or memories, cognitive dissonance, trauma split, unforgiveness, detrimental expectations, victimization, codependent enslavement, ego attachment, fears & all fear states, worries, anxieties, guilt, blame, shame, unresolved grief and sadness, rage, anger suppressed, obsessed, jealousy, need for control, feeling it should have happened differently, brain hemisphere imbalance, mental and emotional instability, non-beneficial Archetypes, polluted thought patterns, brainwashing, repressed positive emotions, fear of success, value in the body, any limiting religious beliefs, protective guarding, all trapped emotions, heart walls, hidden heart walls, and negative emotion imprints.

The ECM, aka fascia, not only influences body movement but also emotions. Dysfunction in the ECM can cause emotional alteration in the person.[76]

The original ACE (Adverse Childhood Experiences) study was conducted at Kaiser Permanente from 1995 to 1997 with two waves of data collection. Over 17,000 Health Maintenance Organization members from Southern California receiving physical exams completed confidential surveys regarding their childhood experiences and current health status and behaviors. They found that the more adverse childhood experiences, the higher the likelihood of illness later in life.[77,78]

It makes me wonder how much of those childhood traumas, such as child abuse and neglect, are stored in the ECM.

One influential book I recommend is The Body Keeps the Score by Bessel Van Der Kolk. The author did a great job with the stories throughout the book and the concept that our bodies store those memories. I listened to the audiobook version and had to pause and take some breaks here and there as some of the stories were tough to hear. That is my warning if you are a strong empath like me.

The definition of an empath "is the action of understanding, being aware of, being sensitive to, and vicariously experiencing the feelings, thoughts, and experience of another."[79]

An empath is a person who is highly sensitive to the feelings and emotions of others; in a way, they can actually feel what another person is feeling. Judy Dyer has some good books for those wanting to read more about the topic.

"Energetic," refers to energy communication systems within the body and fields around and within the body. One consists of the meridian system and its associated points, like acupoints, central to Traditional Chinese Medicine (TCM).

Research shows that the fascial system (ECM) emits biophotons and adjustable sounds as a means of local and systemic cellular communication.[80]

Collagen within the extracellular matrix is made from a triple helix formation of collagen fibers called tropocollagen. These collagen fibers create a continuous nanotubule network throughout the body that allows for information communication. The collagen network is important in dictating cell behavior.[81]

Glyphosate, chemically called N-phosphonomethyl glycine, is the most widely used biocide (herbicide) on the planet and clinically is a highly toxic poison to humans. Glyphosate is very similar to the amino acid glycine and can insert itself in place of the glycine in collagen.[82,83] I believe this is a major cause of fibromyalgia and inflammation in the ECM. Author Ginevra Liptan discusses the histological changes seen in fibromyalgia patients:

> "Recent biopsy studies using immune-histochemical staining techniques have found increased levels of collagen and inflammatory mediators in the connective tissue surrounding the muscle cells in fibromyalgia patients."[84]

Remember, when feel you are negatively impacted by a toxin, a microorganism or have a challenging organ or tissues in the body, you can use that as your specific focus during the Clear It Template. Being aware of something allows you to clear it.

Other things that would fall into the "Energetic" category are Nadis, subtle energy channels believed to carry prana (vital energy) throughout the body.

Chakras, which consist of seven primary energy centers or points in the body, are believed to be located along the Sushumna Nadi, which are on the midline of the body. Each chakra corresponds to different organs and areas of our body, as shown in picture below.

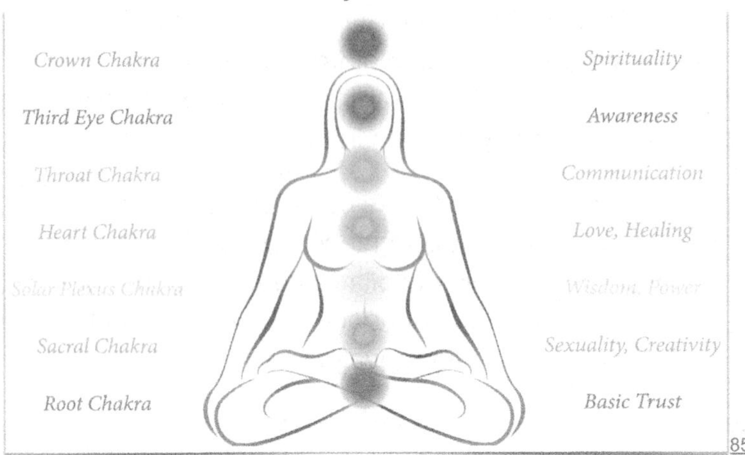

[85]

Dr. Jere Rivera-Dugenio believes that the true energy centers without distortions are called Sha'Ka'Ras., There are 7 primary Sha'Ka'Ras in the body and 15 in total. These Sha'Ka'Ras are part of the Level 2 BioRegenesis grid.

Quantum Morphogenetic Physics recognizes 12 primary Axi-A-Tonal Lines that might have a Traditional Chinese Medicine meridian appearance at first glance, but are different. Dr. Jere Rivera-Dugenio states, "Axi-A-Tonal Lines are points where the rotating, single-axis flash-line sequences from the Seed Crystal Seals cross over and through each other to form 12 primary vertical flowlines within the body."[51]

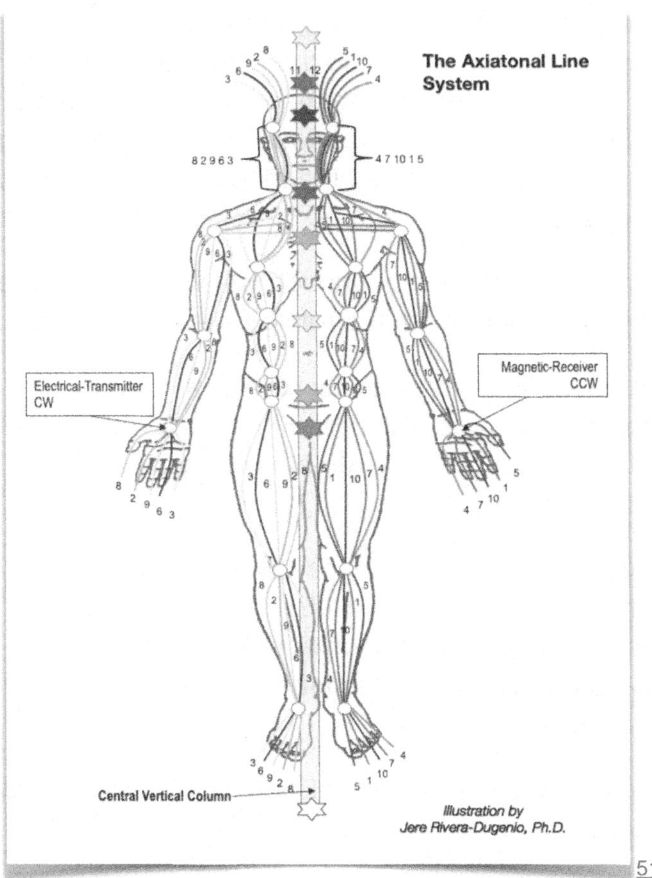

[51]

Fields are also included in the “Energetics” category, as well as the BioRegenesis points taught in Quantum Morphogenetic Physics coursework.

“Spiritual” refers to and is not limited to the following: hexes, curses, spells, black magic, bad medicine, witchcraft, psychic attacks, psychic infections, psychic laser rays/ships, mind control, negative objects, negative energy patterns, negative thought forms, blocking shields, energetic weapons and other being energies.[42]

The "Environment" refers to anything local in the environment all the way up to the galaxy and cosmic levels, such as EMFs, nature, geopathic stress, social environment, morphic (morphogenetic) fields, anything at home, work, other spaces, other dimensions, Earth, solar, lunar, cosmic energies, and negative astrological influence.

The following is research I thought was interesting and thought-provoking about the related environment category:

On Oct. 30, 2020, Popular Mechanics, a science and technology magazine, published that the Earth keeps pulsating with tiny seismic rumbles every 26 seconds, and no one knows why.[86]

Research published in 2019 has shown that the Earth's Extremely Low Frequency (ELF) electromagnetic resonances, called the Schumann Resonances, are associated with cardioprotection via a creatine kinase release association.[87]

The Schumann Resonance is Earth's natural heartbeat rhythm frequency of 7.83 HZ.[88]

Research published in 2020 showed a clear correlation between Schumann Resonance energy and the number of cardiovascular-related hospital admissions.[89]

Other research published in 2018 by Abdullah Alabdulgader et al. states, "There are studies that indicate that geomagnetic disturbances can exacerbate existing diseases, can lead to cardiac arrhythmias, cardiovascular disease, a significant increase in hospitalization rates for mental disorders, depression, suicide attempts, homicide, and traffic accidents."[90] Essentially saying that the energetic environment around people has a large impact on our health.

Research published in the early 1980s by Lorne K. Direnfeld from Boston University states, "…it is possible that the dominant frequencies of brain waves may be an evolutionary result of the presence and influence of the resonant ELF electromagnetic background of Schumann." Direnfeld L.K. The Genesis of the EEG and its Relation to Electromagnetic Radiation.[91] She is basically saying that the Earth's background energies influence our brain waves and state.

Research published in 2021 by Samantha M. Tracy et al. states, "Our findings suggest that periods of increased solar and geomagnetic activity result in lower WBC, neutrophil, and basophil counts that may contribute to slight immune suppression."[92] To summarize, the Sun and Earth's energies impact human immune system function.

Research published in 2019 by Jing-Yau Tang et al. states, "These results indicate that a Schumann resonance frequency of 7.83 Hz can inhibit the growth of cancer cells and that using a specific frequency type can lead to more effective growth inhibition."[93]

The research above makes a strong point that humans are impacted by the energetic environment around them. This is why it is critical to comprehend and include it in the Clear It Template.

> "If you want to find the secrets of the universe, think in terms of energy, frequency, and vibration."
> ~Nikola Tesla

At the time of publication, there are two different websites where you can view current data about the Schumann

Resonance:

- http://sosrff.tsu.ru/ shows a time of 6 hours ahead of UTC zone (Coordinated Universal Time). It is in Russian, but you can still understand the data based on the chart provided
- http://www.vlf.it/cumiana/last-marconi-multistrip-slow.jpg shows the last 5-6 days

Research Michał Zimecki published in 2006 regarding the moon (lunar) cycle states, "Human and animal physiology are subject to seasonal, lunar, and circadian rhythms." "The lunar cycle has an impact on human reproduction, in particular fertility, menstruation, and birth rate." "Admittance to hospitals and emergency units because of various causes (cardiovascular and acute coronary events, variceal hemorrhage, diarrhea, urinary retention) correlated with moon phases. In addition, other events associated with human behavior, such as traffic accidents, crimes, and suicides, appeared to be influenced by the lunar cycle."[94] Women's menstrual cycles have always been the same length as a moon (lunar) cycle, but the above lists many more things connected to the moon's cycle.

"Time" is a complex topic. In Part H, it is described as the past, present, future, alternate time spheres, etc. It exists as a dimension as well as a philosophical and cultural construct. Time can be a noun, a verb, or an adjective, depending on how we use it, which adds to its intrigue and reflects the multifaceted nature of this fundamental concept.

Physicists typically define time as a measurement of change and as a measurement of energy or force in motion. The *Analysis and Assessment of Gateway Process* document, now declassified by the CIA, states:

> "...human consciousness can, with enough practice, move beyond the dimension of time-space and interface with other energy systems in other dimensions..."[44]

The more you process and explore all the different aspects of time, the greater the results you will achieve with the Clear It Template.

In my work, I have uncovered many "Antennas" and "Receivers" within the human body. These words seem to be used interchangeably at times.

"Antennas" are primarily responsible for transmitting or receiving information. Traditional science would mainly say that antennas transmit and receive electromagnetic waves. Transverse electromagnetism consists of sine and cosine waves. Scalar energy exists as well and is sometimes referred to as longitudinal waves.

At the time of this writing, I have found with my own testing that there are a total of 12,222 different antennas in and around each of us. Published research by Martin Blank and Reba Goodman from Columbia University in 2011 titled *DNA is a fractal antenna in electromagnetic fields*. The authors conclude the following:

> "The wide frequency range of interaction with EMF is the functional characteristic of a fractal antenna, and DNA appears to possess the two structural characteristics of fractal antennas, electronic conduction and self-symmetry. These properties contribute to greater reactivity of DNA with EMF in the environment, and the DNA damage could

> account for increases in cancer epidemiology, as well as variations in the rate of chemical evolution in early geologic history."[95]

I believe more and more antennas within and around the body will be identified in the coming century.

"Receivers" process the signal the antenna receives and convert it into usable information by the body. At the time of this writing, I believe from my own testing that there are 134,333 different receivers in and around each of us.

The human being is truly amazing, and science continues to make new discoveries daily. For instance, we now know the heart has its own brain cells. Researchers have found that the heart has a nervous system containing around 40,000 neurons called sensory neurites. This extensive and complex neural network has been characterized as a brain on the heart or heart-brain.[96]

PART J

(j) **Related to every combination, in the proper order, as many times as needed.**

Going back to the Part D example story…

> "For example, imagine John Doe getting off the phone with his boss, who just told him that he has been unexpectedly promoted to a higher position and will now make double his previous salary. John is ecstatic and decides to go for a joy ride in his car to celebrate. Ten minutes into his drive, his girlfriend calls him and tells him she does not want to be in a relationship with him anymore. At that very moment, a drunk driver crashes into John's car, hitting him so hard he goes unconscious,

and an ambulance takes him to the hospital."

"Related to every combination, in the proper order, as many times as needed" refers to every piece of a series of collective events in a specific order. The emotion of surprise came first, followed by the feeling of joy following the unexpected raise and the connection to a person (being his boss). Then, changing to the connection with his car and joy riding with the change of environment. Followed by a phone call from his girlfriend.

The point is that there was an order in which the events took place. We repeat the connection of all these elements in order "as many times as needed," so nothing is missed.

PART K

(k) **Including all**: consciousness and unconsciousness states, ETHUR, SP°, scaylons, scalar points, levels, dimensions, bodies, Eukatharista body, morphogenetic crystal body, mind, morphic fields, BPR, Sha'Ka'Ras, crystal seals, field, field Generator, UM-Shaddh-Eie, DNA, intron DNA, body encoding system, AzurA dish, holograms, sacred geomancies, and light symbol codes.

"Consciousness and unconsciousness states" wording and intention is to cover all levels of consciousness. There are different types of consciousness defined by neuroscience-based upon what areas of the brain are activated and what brain waves the brain is predominately firing via an EEG. I would not limit types of consciousness to just what mainstream neuroscience identifies and measures. You can also include different levels of consciousness, from someone being stressed out to being euphoric to praying or meditating or even being on psychedelic substances.

Unconsciousness refers to sleeping, dreaming, comas, being drugged out or passed out from alcohol and general anesthesia.

The majority of Part K wording I have included comes from Quantum Morphogenetic Physics at BioRegenesisAcademy.org. The intention is to cover the smallest particle or molecule up to the biggest of the body anatomically. In my current view, Quantum Morphogenetic Physics has the most detailed explanations.

Although the below can feel overwhelming or confusing, especially the first time reading this, it is critical to include in this book and in the Clear It Template, as this is the basis on which the body is created.

"ETHUR," also written as E-TH-UR, is the first original state of pre-substance that is encoded with the Base-12 mathematical encryption. The Base-12 BioRegenesis Grid comprises 12 geleziac radiation spheres composed of E-TH-UR.[51]

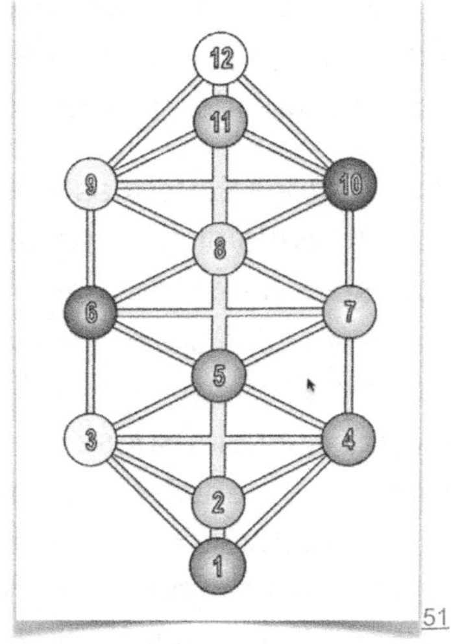

[51]

The Base-12 BioRegenesis Grid looks similar to the Kabbalistic tree of life, but some distinct differences exist. There are five stages of pre-substance.[20]

Stage 1: Feeling
Stage 2: Emotion
Stage 3: Thought
Stage 4: IDEA-gel
Stage 5: IDEA crystals

"SP°" stands for Source Particle and is also called the original Source Particle. This Source Particle unit then divides into Source Particle Negative (SP-ve) units and Source Particle Positive (SP+ve) units that are interwoven units of bi-polar light energy emission generating electromagnetic, scalar standing waves.[25]

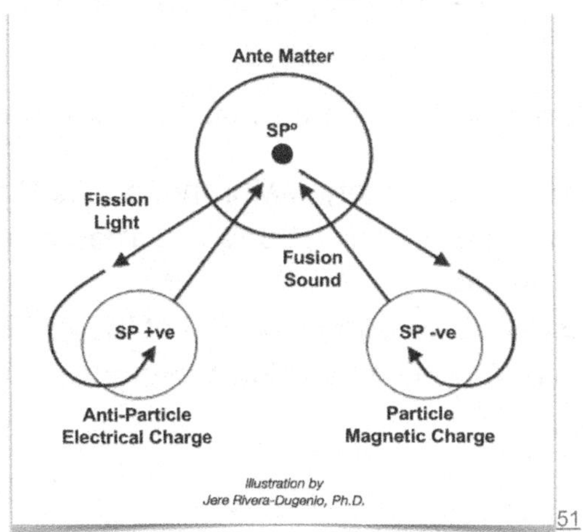

[51]

Mainstream science says that electromagnetic energy is a fundamental form of energy that permeates our universe. This energy is composed of electric and magnetic fields that oscillate together, creating waves. What is missed is that the Source Particle, which is scalar energy, is the parent to SP-ve, the magnetic charge, and SP+ve, the electrical charge. In other words, scalar energy is the parent of electromagnetic energy.[51]

Source Particles are the smallest units of energy that form matter and anti-matter. 800 million Source Particles equal one proton.[51]

"Scaylons" synthesize light-sound, fission-fusion energy units known as Source Particle.[97] These "Scaylons" then group with other "Scaylons" to form dimensionalized crystalline structures of energy that exist as the base morphogenetic (form-holding) templates behind and within all matter forms, particles, and consciousness. These structures modulate the speed, angles, and patterns of the SP° configurations, acting like a sort of organizational software. Scaylons can also be referred to as subatomic particles.[51]

Scalar points refer to electro-tonal flash-line sequences.[51]

"Levels" refer to the Quantum Morphogenetic Physics definitions of levels, in which there are three levels of the BioRegenesis Grid.
Level-1: Base-12 BioRegenesis Grid of the INTERNAL TEMPLAR along with the Shields & Signets.[51]

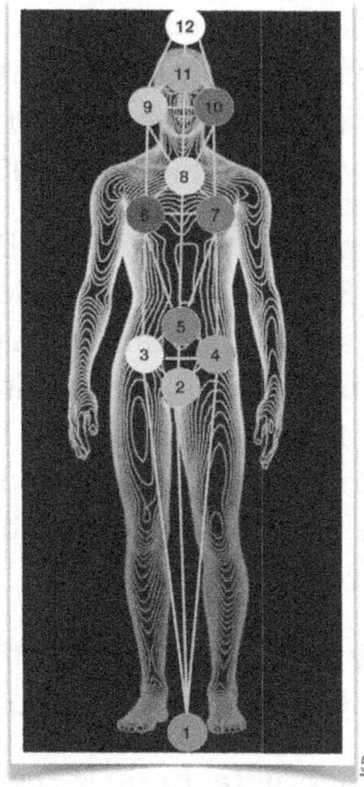

[51]

Level-2 BioRegenesis Crystal Seals Grid and Sha'Ka'Ras. In the human body, the 15 primary Star Crystal Seals exist between each of the 15 Sha'Ka'Ras on the central BioRegenesis Line (or central body current or central vertical current). They serve as frequency seals that open or close the flow of wave spectra and frequency bands from one Harmonic Universe of consciousness to another.[51]

The Axi-A-Tonal Lines create the web-work of energy upon which the BioRegenesis Grid Level-3 Diodic and Miodics Points and DNA manifest.[51]

Dimensions refer to a full frequency sphere or full cycle of a Flash-line Sequence within a morphogenetic field. Think of them as dimensional spheres. There are 15-dimensional Time Matrices within which manifestation can be experienced. The higher the dimensional sphere, the faster the Source Particle phasing, the higher the oscillation, and the lower the vibration. Each one of the 15 dimensions contains 12 Primary Sub-frequency Rings.[51]

Bodies refer to a collection of Aah-JhA' Body, Spirit Body, Rasha Body, Light Body, and Physical Body. The Spirit and Rasha Bodies are eternal, and the Light and Physical Bodies are finite. The Aah-JhA' creates the Spirit Body, the Spirit Body creates the Rasha Body, the Rasha Body creates the Light Body, and the Light Body creates the Physical Body. The Rasha body is considered a significant link in the chain.[51]

Eukatharista body is the collection of all the bodies into one. It is the Living Creation-Manifestation Matrix.[51]

The **morphogenetic crystal body** is Scaylon Codes within our multidimensional structure, also known as the Source Particle Grid. The morphogenetic crystal body field governs the form of matter manifestation. Everything has a morphogenetic crystal body structure. This is akin to the morphogenetic skeleton upon which our physical and subtle bodies are constructed.[51]

The **Mind** is an immaterial and non-physical thing that experiences consciousness while the body carries out its instructions. Most think of the brain and mind as the same thing, but I like to see them as separate things.

Morphic fields refer to Part T. Also known as morphogenetic fields; they exist as scalar energy fields of inter-woven Source Particles. The morphogenetic field of a being exists as part of the larger morphogenetic field of the planet.[51]

BPR refers to the Base Pulse Rhythm, the cumulative sum of the frequency vibration of the core Encryption Lattice at any given moment. It can be visualized as the core heartbeat or foundational rhythm.[51]

Sha'Ka'Ras refer to the multidimensional energy source system, which consists of 15 primary Sha'Ka'Ras, nine of them located within the physical body structure and six in the bioenergetic field. Sha'Ka'Ras draw energy in from and transmit energy into the Unified Fields of each Dimension. Each Sha'Ka'Ra corresponds to a level of the Auric Field and one Axi-A-Tonal Line. These are essentially our inner stargate system and the key to Inscension. Sha'Ka'Ra is part of Level 2 BioRegenesis Grid.[51]

Crystal seals are groups of 3-dimensional SP° scalar wave composites that regulate the rate of SP° phasing to create the base structures upon which dimensionalization is formed. As mentioned in the above "Levels," they are frequency seals between each Sha'Ka'Ra, and there are 15 primary ones.[51]

The picture below illustrates 15 primary Sha'Ka'Ras indicated with the letter "S" and associated number. It also shows the 15 primary crystal seals indicated with the letters "C" and "MC" along with their associated number.

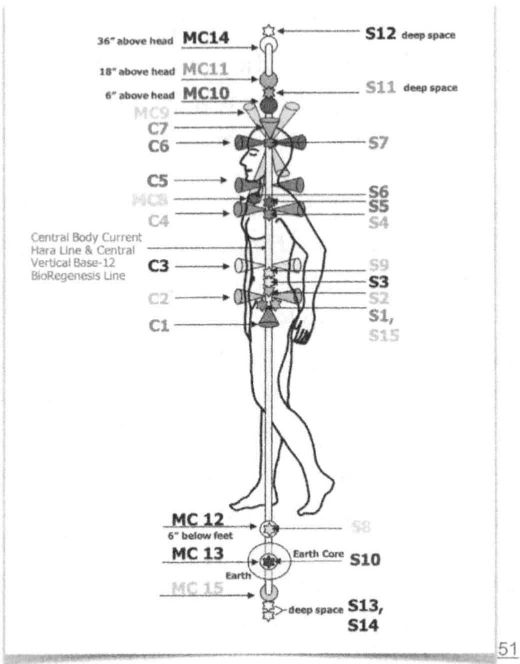

[51]

Field refers to a sphere-shaped area around the body that is part of the sending and receiving messages from the environment.

Field Generator refers to a point near the solar plexus that creates a field around the human body.

UM-Shaddh-Eie is located at the bottom of the pelvis and is the core template upon which the core of our DNA templates are built. This core template runs the Axi-A-Tonal Lines and meridian lines system.[51]

DNA is the instruction manual that tells your body how to build and function. Friedrich Miescher discovered DNA in the late 1860s without knowing its importance. In 1953, James Watson and Francis Crick discovered the double-helix structure of DNA. Unfortunately, Rosalind Franklin's work was never given any credit. Watson was shown one of Rosalind's key X-ray diffraction patterns without her knowledge, and Crick was shown one of her progress reports. With Rosalynn's X-ray crystallography information, Watson and Crick theorized that the DNA had to be a double helix shape. They later won the Nobel Prize for this discovery.[98]

Science states that DNA is a twisted ladder formation known as the double helix consisting of repeating nucleotides, recognizing one DNA strand. Research Giulia Biffi et al. from the University of Cambridge published in 2013 shows that a four-stranded DNA structure exists.[99]

At this moment, I believe humans hold a 12-strand DNA template,[97] and some even hold the potential for 24 or even 48. Time will tell as science advances its knowledge in this area. As Wayne Gretzky has said, do not skate to where the puck is, but skate to where the puck is going.

Intron DNA refers to the non-coding sequences found within genes. These are specific frequency patterns that have been disassembled. Science typically calls this junk DNA. However, we can learn to unlock this intron DNA, which would in turn unleash true human potential.

The **body encoding system** refers to a system in a human body that is responsible for gathering information from the Morphogenetic field around the physical body. This information is then gathered, interpreted, and shared in order for the human body to be able to exist in materialized form.

AzurA dish refers to a slightly curved disk-shaped receptor located just in front of the thymus area. This receptor can change angles like a satellite dish.

Holograms – Quantum morphogenetic field physics proposes that the human body is a holographic projection of consciousness created upon a holographic design of organized units of consciousness.[51]

Sacred geomancies are specific patterns of conscious scalar standing energy waves that give consciousness its individualized form in time. They are the building blocks the Source-Mind uses in its processes of creation. They are sets of mathematical and geometrical principles that serve as the blueprints for how Sub-Quantum Particles (SPs) should be arranged in any given structure or system.[51]

Light symbol codes refer to patterns of electro-tonal energy composed of specific SP° configurations that create frequencies and spectrums of multidimensional sound and light.[51]

PART L

- (l) **Along with all** active vows, commitments, contracts, and agreements.

"Vows, commitments, contracts, and agreements" all involve promises and obligations with distinct nuances. "Vows" are the most personal, often emotional declarations made to oneself or another. They hold a deep significance, carrying weight beyond formal rules. "Commitments," while serious, are broader. They encompass intentional choices to act in a certain way, often tied to values or responsibilities.

“Contracts and agreements,” on the other hand, are formal arrangements. They outline specific terms and conditions, often with legal implications.

“Vows” bind our hearts, “commitments” guide our actions, and “contracts” ensure shared expectations.

There are things that people have said or agreed to in the past that, when remembered or become aware of, would not be agreed to anymore. It is critical to clear and release those.

This also encapsulates “vows, commitments, contracts, and agreements” that influence you that you were not a part of making. This is focusing on what is active and not positive in your life.

Part M

- (m) **If any hitchhikers have not completed** their chosen life path, take them to the farthest depths of darkness right now to complete their life path.

While this is not typically needed, I have found it to come up a few times, so I include it in the Clear It Template.

If everything comes from source, then everything is part of source. If a spirit’s destiny is to create and experience darkness, source will only turn it back into light once it has fulfilled that path.

That is why the phrase “take them to the farthest depth of darkness right now to complete their life path” is written. Remember, the whole point is to release any detrimental, harmful, interfering, distorting, and manipulating energies from you so your true self can just "be."

PART N

(n) **Lock into everything associated**: Chemical, Physical, Environmental, Mental, Emotional, Spiritual.

As I wrote in Part D, every event is connected to other events, as well as emotions, people, etc. The purpose is to connect all associated things from every possible category to allow our bodies to release and clear them. When you realize that everything is connected you look at life differently.

Please refer to Part D for a more detailed example of how multiple events, people, emotions, etc., can all be connected to one overall event.

Please refer to Part I for definitions of "Chemical, Physical, Environmental, Mental, Emotional, Spiritual."

PART O

(o) **Deleting, transmuting, and removing (everything)** from all consciousness and unconsciousness states, ETHUR, SP°, scaylons, scalar points, levels, dimensions, bodies, Eukatharista body, morphogenetic crystal body, mind, morphic fields, BPR, Sha'Ka'Ras, crystal seals, field, field Generator, UM-Shaddh-Eie, DNA, intron DNA, body encoding system, AzurA dish, holograms, sacred geomancies, and light symbol codes.

This is a repeat of Part K except Part K referred to "including all" of the above. Where Part O refers to "deleting, transmuting, and removing from all."

The words "deleting, transmuting, and removing" are also very intentional, and I would recommend revisiting the beginning of Part G if you need a reminder about them.

Please refer to Part K for the definitions and explanations for the following: "consciousness and unconsciousness states, ETHUR, SP°, scaylons, scalar points, levels, dimensions, bodies, Eukatharista body, morphogenetic crystal body, mind, morphic fields, BPR, Sha'Ka'Ras, crystal seals, field, field Generator, UM-Shaddh-Eie, DNA, intron DNA, body encoding system, AzurA dish, holograms, sacred geomancies, and light symbol codes."

PART P

(p) **Releasing (everything)** all limiting factors, attractors, attachments, identification to these patterns & identities, especially given by others, and protective guarding.

A "limiting factor" is anything that restricts or prevents something from reaching its full potential. It can be a bottleneck that slows down or stops progress.

An "attractor" is something on or around you that acts like a magnet toward a specific thing or action. For example, imagine that you decided when you were younger that you were going to be just like your father or mother. Now you are subconsciously drawn toward things that would help fulfill that and deterred from things that do not fulfill that. I am not referring to anything related to your soul purpose or passion for your life's mission.

An "attachment" refers to a strong, enduring connection that you form with another person, place, object, or even an idea. This connection involves both cognitive and emotional elements.

“Identification of these patterns & identities” refers to personal, social, and cultural patterns and personal, social, and ideological identities. Personal patterns are recurring thoughts, feelings, and behaviors. Social patterns include your social interactions and your communication style. Cultural patterns are cultural values and practices that provide a sense of belonging and inform your worldview. Personal identities are individual values and characteristics that make you unique, such as your interests, skills, and talents. Social identities usually refer to group affiliations like race, ethnicity, gender, and sexual orientation. Ideological identities are groups you feel affiliated with that are related to politics, religion, or philosophy.

“Especially given by others” refers to getting these patterns and identities from someone outside yourself, such as parents, siblings, uncles, aunts, friends, coworkers, bosses, teachers, babysitters, etc.

Some examples of statements that can influence your identity:

- You are such a wild kid.
- You are just like your brother.
- You are so dumb and lazy.
- You can’t help it. You are bipolar just like your grandmother.
- Depression runs in the family. You are going to be depressed too.

“Protective guarding” refers to any neurological wiring you have created to protect that previously injured area. Since I had knee surgery when I was 17 years old, anytime someone would get close to my knee, especially a health practitioner, I would start guarding it because it was such a sensitive area. The more repetitive trauma you have to an area, the easier it is to create this "protective guarding."

PART Q

(q) **Collapsing all those energies into the source grid, back into light.**

This critical part of the Clear It Template has significant implications and cannot be missed.

An extremely knowledgeable and fit doctor approached me at the workshop where I first taught the Clear It Template in late 2023. He had knee pain and he could not figure out what was causing it. After testing and listening to my intuition, I told him that whatever his knee pain was from, it was somehow related to the Earth and his connection to the Earth and that he needed to connect the dots. An hour later he returned to me and said he thought he had figured it out. He learned at a seminar in the past that when clearing entities and demons, he should send them to the middle of Earth. He realized that when I said it was somehow connected to Earth, it had to do with all the entities and demons he sent to Earth that Earth was still holding onto. He said that he sent all the hitchhikers into Earth back into light. After he did that, all his knee pain disappeared that he was experiencing. This is another example of how our body or soul communicates with us through physical symptoms to get our attention. The doctor shared with the entire audience what had happened and that his knee pain disappeared.

After that doctor shared his Aha moment and instant

results, I had another doctor friend tell me that he took a seminar a while ago about clearing entities from people by this repetitive swiping motion along the person's body to release the entity from the person. The person's wrist and arm pain disappeared as my practitioner friend performed this clearing motion. As my friend drove home from the seminar, he started having the same pains as the person he just worked on. He realized that he had released the entity from the person, and it then attached to him.

After that doctor told me that story, it reminded me of a book I read a few years ago called "Reweaving the Fabric of Your Reality" by Maureen J. St. Germain. It is a shorter book originally published in 2004 and gives a few different types of clearing. One of the types was called the "Cutting Ceremony," which involved taking a stainless-steel knife or sword and cutting through the air and space around your body. When trying to disconnect them from your body, the hitchhikers will attach to someone else or reattach to you. I remember reading that book thinking the whole topic of entities was significant but not feeling like the solutions offered were impactful.

The takeaway point is that all the energies we release, especially hitchhikers, must be returned to light. Otherwise, these beings will reattach back to you or someone else.

While reading "**Collapsing all those energies into the source grid, back into light.**" I visualize all the energies released being gathered into a cloud of energy starting at the head area and gathering the rest of the energies up as the cloud moves towards the feet. I then breathe in and, on the exhale, visualize the cloud leaving the feet area and being sent into the source grid.

As discussed in Part K, technically, all light comes from source particles first. If you prefer you could change this to "Collapsing all those energies into the source grid, back into source particles."

PART R

(r) ***Reversing all ill effects and filling all voids with source love, light, and oscillations.***

Unwanted or harmful effects are what I refer to as "**ill effects**," and those can happen after a trauma, a stressor, etc. "**Reversing all ill effects**" is to bring something back into its optimal state before the event altered the person, tissues, and energies.

When energy is removed from an area it leaves behind a void or a space. "***Filling all voids with source love, light, and oscillations***" is intentionally not leaving that space empty. The space could be filled with the same thing that left it or something else. In order to avoid allowing another unwelcome energy to take over the space, I intentionally fill it with "**source love, light, and oscillations**."

"**Love**" is a great thing to fill a void with. I am not referring to lustful love but the actual state of love. As with the whole Clear It Template, use words that make the most sense to you. You could replace "**love**" with joy, peace, or enlightenment if you would like.

The word "**oscillations**" is often used interchangeably with vibrations, but as Dr. Jere Rivera-Dugenio states, these words have entirely different meanings. In physics, vibration is energy holding, which is energy contraction. When you have high vibrations or are highly vibratory, you are dense. Oscillation refers to energy expansion. The higher the oscillations, the higher the energy expansion. Vibration and oscillation exist in direct proportion to each other. As vibration increases (energy holding), oscillation decreases (energy expenditure).[51]

PART S

(s) **Repeat as many times as needed.**

When creating a health protocol for a patient, there is a particular order in which one needs to proceed to maximize the benefit. I think of it as peeling away layers of an onion. For instance, one does not want to immediately attempt to eliminate pathogens or push detox hard if the body's drainage pathways are clogged. That is equivalent to putting more things into a sink that is already clogged. The first step is to unclog the sink. The same is true from an energetic release standpoint. Early on when I was doing clearings, I was working through what was first to clear, linking with all the attached associations and clearing them. I would then do the next item and read through the Clear It Template. It hit me one day that I should just say, "**Repeat as many times as needed**" at the end of reading this so it repeats subconsciously. Basically, I was able to put the template on auto-pilot so that I did not have to keep reciting it. This sped up the clearing process, so I did not have to continue reading the Clear It Template repeatedly.

PART T

(t) **Delete, transmute, and remove all mutations, interference, manipulations, and distortions.**

The beginning of Part G contains the specifics on why the words "**Delete, transmute, and remove**" are used.

A "**mutation**" is generally defined as a change in the DNA sequence of an organism.[100]

Mainstream science says that "**mutations**" are permanent. I think of the word "**mutation**" as an alteration of any part or field of the body at that moment. It is not limited to only a DNA or chromosome mutation, nor must it be permanent.

Mainstream science still thinks that DNA holds the blueprint for us. At the time of writing this book, I tend to believe that DNA is more of an antenna and pulls in information from the field around us.

Rupert Sheldrake has researched and written books on the topic of morphic resonance. He references morphic fields within that topic, also called morphogenetic fields. He defines a morphic field as a non-physical field that surrounds and interacts with living systems, influencing their form and behavior across time and space. He proposes that these fields hold a memory of past forms and interactions, allowing them to guide the development and behavior of similar systems in the past. When the first version of his book was published, the journal Nature called it "the best candidate for the burning there has been for many years."[101]

My ears always perk up when I hear mainstream science wants to do a book burning on a topic. That usually tells me there is some truth to that subject, and they do not want us to know.

The word "field" in the morphic field refers to scalar energy, rather than electromagnetic field energy, which can potentially be confusing from a mainstream science perspective. At some point, there might be a benefit to using an alternate word to avoid confusion.

"Morphic Resonance is destined to become one of the landmarks in the history of biology. It is rare to find so profound a book so lucidly written." ~Bruce H. Lipton, PhD[102]

"**Interference**" refers to anything that hinders or obstructs something. In a simplified manner, I think of static when listening to a radio station. There is interference from your radio receiving the radio tower signal. Our bodies have many receivers and antennas on them, so any interference that impacts any one of those many receivers and antennas can be detrimental to our overall health optimization.

"**Manipulation**" refers to any subtle or overt deceptive influence over you. This can involve being fed inaccurate, withholding, or distorting information and facts. This can also include emotional manipulation, which involves playing on another person's emotions, such as guilt, pity, fear, or love, to influence them deceptively.

"**Distortions**" refer to any deviation from an ideal or norm, intentionally or unintentionally. This can involve but is not limited to, the physical body, the fields around us, our environment, including Earth, and even pure water. I assume many things within our reality have distortions unless proven otherwise.

Part U

(u) **Delete, transmute, and remove all detrimental**

external energies and shift my energy to avoid being impacted.

The beginning of Part G contains the specifics on why the words "**Delete, transmute, and remove**" are used.

Detrimental external energies refer to anything outside of you that is unwanted or negative being sent your way. Early on, when I discovered more and more of these detrimental types of energies, I got angry and wanted to battle them. My intention became to reflect and exponentially magnify all harmful energies back to where they came from without them knowing it was me reflecting that energy back. I would put up an infinite amount of protective shielding in an attempt to prevent any impact from other harmful energies and put a cloak up to distract the energies.

Needless to say, I was spending a lot of time and effort trying to figure out how to "win over" these "**detrimental external energies**." Fast forward, I discovered that it only increased the energies to what seemed like an unending amount of evil in the world. Then, one morning in my quiet time, I had the fleeting thought that you do not wage a war without the other side by fighting back. Opposing energies want nothing more than to engage in a fight against you, knowing that this will feed into the duality and polarity of this world. I decided not to fight and focus my attention inward on myself.

In Chapter 3, I discussed the idea that everything is energy. Waging war is not the answer if those "**detrimental external energies**" will always exist. Therefore, I decided to instead focus on shifting my the angular rotation of particle spin of my cells so that the energies do not impact me.

I imagine you may be wondering what angular rotation of particle spin is. Imagine you shoot a bow and arrow at a target. Let's say the target is just a thin piece of paper, and the moment before the arrow hits the target, I rotate the target 90 degrees. That arrow will sail by the target because there is nothing but the width of the piece of paper for the arrow to get now. To take it one step further, when the angle is rotated at 90 degrees, the actual target disappears. The dimension above and below us is accessed when our angular rotation particle spin is moved 90 degrees, along with subsequent dimensions.

It is interesting to think about this regarding EMFs, which is technically EMR (electromagnetic radiation). An increasingly growing number of people have sensitivities to WIFI, Bluetooth, cell phones, etc. Those people who do not experience any symptoms and do not feel what a small percentage of people can feel and experience think that that group is crazy. It is always easier to make fun of something you have yet to experience.

In Drunvalo Melchizedek's book The Ancient Secret of the Flower of Life Volume 2, he mentions that during his meditations electrical things around him would stop working. In one meditation, he caused the light switch above his head to blow up and catch fire. He then realized that he could shift his energy so that the electrical fields around him were unaffected. After that, he said he no longer had any issues with electronics.

After reading that book, I started thinking about times I had affected electrical devices. One time, when I was presenting a webinar online to 1000 people, I completely killed the internet along with my backup cell phone connection. Toward the end of the webinar, my energy got so high and intense that I short-circuited the internet. It took 15 minutes to get it reconnected.

I also can feel a lot of various types of energies, including WIFI, Bluetooth, and hitchhikers on people. I decided to alter my energy so that these chaotic types of energies do not impact me anymore. Before shifting my energy, I would feel a buzzing type feeling in my head when within 20 feet of a WIFI router.

There are some interesting things Drunvalo Melchizedek presents in his books, but I would caution against his Mer-Ka-Ba technique, as you do not want to phase lock your Mer-Ka-Ba at the wrong spin speed, which is what he teaches. I recommend following Dr. Jere Rivera-Dugenio's Merkaba information for optimal speed and spin.

Research was done on 114 people who were told they were exposed to non-native EMFs. The number of people saying they experienced symptoms from the non-native EMFs was shocking. The participants later found it was a complete shame study, and they were never exposed any of the participants to EMFs.[103]

This is a great example showing the power of our minds and what they can create. The above study shows that psychosomatic exists. Psychosomatic refers to physical symptoms influenced by a person's mental or emotional state.

I bring this up to illustrate that we have the ability to shift our energy. This is not presented to judge whether EMFs are harmful or not.

Some "**detrimental external energies**" that I have found to have an impact are Saturn, the black cube of Saturn, black rock, the moon (artificial and real), Nibiru (aka planet X), CERN, HAARP, HAARP-like devices, NexRads, Baal, and Baphomet.

PART V

(v) **Delete, transmute, and remove all energies being extracted and shift my energy not to allow.**

The beginning of Part G contains the specifics on why the words "**Delete, transmute, and remove**" are used.

Suppose you put air in your car tire, but you don't realize that your tire has a nail in it. The air does not stay at the proper pressure because of the air being extracted via the nail hole. You will only maintain the air inside the tire once you plug that hole or replace the tire.

Your body produces your weight in ATP every single day.[104] ATP is the energy currency of the body from a biochemical perspective. If detrimental forces exist within your body or your field, they are extracting energy from you, which prevents you from reaching an optimal state of health.

As an example I think of the 1999 film The Matrix when they show the humans stored in pods, and the machine is siphoning the humans' energy for itself. Refer to Part U for more details on shifting your energy.

PART W

(w) **Delete, transmute, and remove all fulfilled and non-**

beneficial: unhealthy commitments, vows, contracts, agreements, and soul agreements.

The beginning of Part G contains the specifics on why the words "**Delete, transmute, and remove**" are used.

The following parts use "unhealthy commitments, contracts, and agreements:" Part F, Part G, Part L, and Part AA.

"Unhealthy commitments" refer to detrimental agreements or pledges to do something in the future.

"Vows" refer to solemn promises or assertions that bind a person to an act, service, or condition.

"Contracts" refer to a binding agreement between two or more parties.

"Agreements" refer to an arrangement, compact, treaty, or executed contract.

"Soul agreements" are pre-birth arrangements made between you and the creator or you and another soul. The agreement could include experiences, lessons learned, challenges to overcome, situations faced, or souls you encounter in a lifetime.

You will notice there are overlaps of meaning within the words above. By using multiple words with similar meanings, I am ensuring I am covering all my bases to clear as much as I can in one reading of the template. I always err on the side of having more than less. It is better to put more words and phrases into the template rather than less because if anything is missed for your particular need, your results will not be optimal.

These unhealthy and "non-beneficial commitments, vows, contracts, agreements, and soul agreements" are being ended due to their harmful nature or the fact that they have been fulfilled or no longer need to exist.

PART X

(x) **Return to when every combination, in the proper order, as many times needed, had no interference, distortions, or manipulations, and bring them forward to now and hold.**

Remember the Part D example?

> "For example, imagine John Doe getting off the phone with his boss, who just told him that he has been unexpectedly promoted and will now make double his previous salary. John is ecstatic and decides to go for a joy ride in his car to celebrate. Ten minutes into his drive, his girlfriend calls him and says she does not want to be in a relationship with him anymore. At that very moment, a drunk driver crashes into John's car, hitting him so hard he goes unconscious, and an ambulance takes him to the hospital."

The Part D example has quite the sequence of events and connections to emotions, people, and events that occur in a specific order.

Not only does the Clear It Template release what is attached to you, but this part helps to unwind all the detrimental and unhealthy changes and alterations that have occurred since the traumas.

Since the inception of your soul's existence, you have accumulated traumas and baggage throughout many lifetimes. The goal is to bring your current physical body and all your other energies to its original state of perfection.

Traumas and baggage have been accumulated and occurred in a specific order and the Clear It Template goes back through all those pieces "**in the proper order**" and repeats "**as many times as needed**." This will ensure that you move back into your true, unaltered state.

Refer to Part T for descriptions of what "**interference, distortions, or manipulations**" mean.

Part Y

(y) **Restore and anchor both polarities and all four cardinal directions in everything.**

I learned this from Peter Seymour Howe, who got it from the late Dr. Bob Marshall. When he explained it to me, I found that polarities and cardinal directions are impactful to add to the Clear It Template.

A magnet contains one side with a negative charge and the opposite side with a positive charge. Traditional theory on magnetic fields says that a magnet holds just one field.

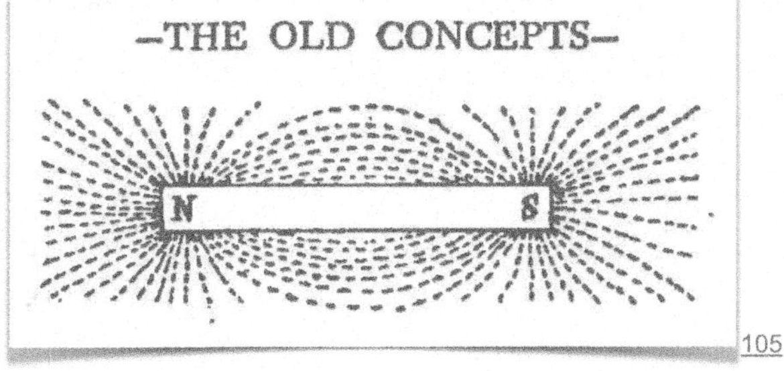

105

In 1936, Albert Roy Davis discovered that magnetism is composed of two fields rather than one. These energies are not static but moving. He also found a difference between north-pole energy and south-pole energy. Furthermore, he discovered that where the north-pole and south-pole energies meet in the middle, there is what is called the Bloch wall, which has no magnetism. The Bloch wall is typically a tiny area.

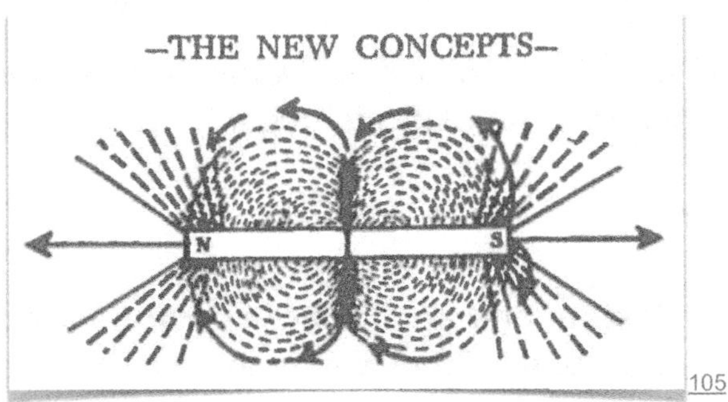

105

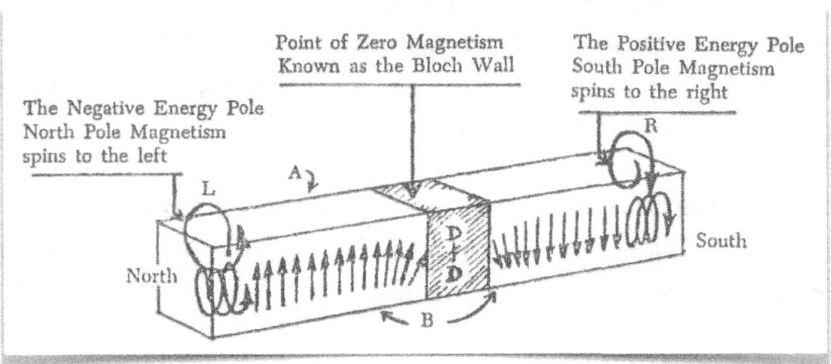

105

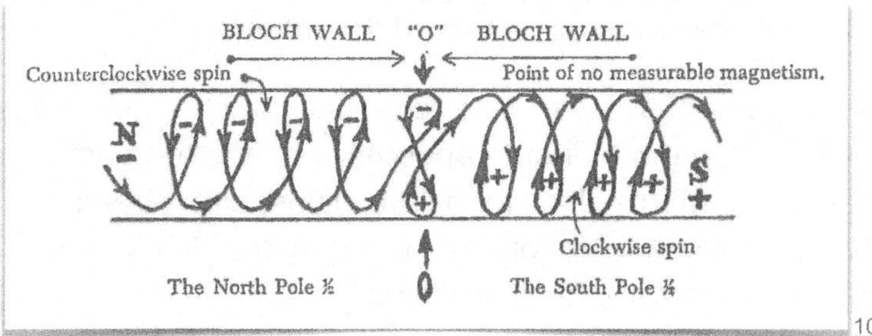

105

Albert Roy Davis discovered that the Earth and humans have a magnetic field containing positive and negative polarity as well. The polarities can get altered by many things including environmental stressors.

Dr. Bob Marshall said the electromagnetic nature of our bodies is highly sensitive to directionality. By directionality, he meant the cardinal directions: north, east, south, and west. In order to visualize this, imagine the four directions of a compass. Restoring both polarities within the body and all four cardinal directions is essential. This helps balance the body, the fields, and all its elements.

When reading "**Restore and anchor both polarities and all four cardinal directions in everything,**" I typically close my eyes and visualize the four compass directions moving away from my body simultaneously as I breathe air out.

PART Z

(z) **Shift the time spheres to reflect the changes made right now**, including the past, the present, the future, this life, all past lives, all probable selves, alternate time spheres, other incarnations, and parallel universes and dimensions.

Part H has more details on the different times.

The purpose of this part is to reflect all the changes made from this moment to instantaneously impact "the past, the present, the future, this life, all past lives, all probable selves, alternate time spheres, other incarnations, and parallel universes and dimensions."

In order to envision this as being possible, it is helpful to disregard linear timeline thinking. Time is a mental construct our brains use to create parameters (past, present future) around events in order make sense of our reality. All you truly have is now, so if you change the now, which the Clear It Template does, then it changes all time.

PART AA

(aa) **"What a great experience, releasing all** hitchhikers, perverse parasitic unhealthy cords, energies, attachments, holograms, fabrications, and beings; manipulations, mutations, distortions, traumas, previous and current unhealthy commitments, contracts, and agreements; body portals, environmental portals, protective guarding, and related energies, all times. **COMPLETED!** (stamped). **Filled with source love, light, and oscillations."**

Imagine there is a library that has documented everything that has happened in your existence, such as every thought, word, deed, event, and emotion. Some people refer to this as the Akashic records. According to Quantum Morphogenetic Physics, there are two additional record-holding areas called the Ecoushic and Rei-ShAic.[51]

When reading this, I envision two librarians who can help write in the Akashic, Ecoushic, and Rei-ShAic records. I imagine one of them pulling the books holding information about me from the shelves, writing in them, and releasing everything mentioned above. I am grateful for all that I am releasing and writing, as there is no need for any anger or harmful emotions to carry. After the books have been written in, I see myself with a large stamper that says "**COMPLETED**" and stamp it on the page. That is my way of closing the loop of what has happened to avoid repeating it.

If voids are created from this process, I "**fill with source love, light, and oscillations**." See Part R for more details on "**love, light**, **and oscillations**."

Part BB

(bb) **Reset, realign, and optimize energy and energy flow to the clearing and create coherence with the energies around me.**

"**Reset**" means returning to the original state before any alterations, distortions, mutations, or interference occur.

"**Realign**" means to bring your body and fields back into a balanced state.

"**Optimize**" refers to bringing your body and fields into an ideal healthy state.

"**Energy flow**" includes the energy moving through all the different parts of the body detailed in Part K, including the Base-12 BioRegenesis Grid, the Sha'Ka'Ras, the Axi-A-Tonal Lines, and meridians.

After "**clearing**" and releasing everything that the Clear It Template includes, it is critical to re-establish the proper energy movement in and around the body.

Also, realize that “**create coherence with the energies around me**” is critical as you will often be more hyper-aware of things that feel “off” around you after you release what was distorting your perspective. Everyone has his or her own journey to walk, and it is not about “fixing” the world with this methodology, but about working on yourself by expanding your consciousness. “**Creating coherence with the energies around me**” will instantly bring peace to you within your environment.

“**Coherence**” refers to integrating all environmental and bodily elements, producing a coherent and balanced energetic state. You can also think of it as consciousness united. An incoherent state is like having a sliver under your skin or one sole of a shoe thicker than another one under your feet.

PART CC

(cc) **Adjust my Merkaba spin to the most appropriate eternal ratio and spin speed and hold for as long as is beneficial.**

In ancient Judaism, Merkabah refers to the chariot throne of God described in the Book of Ezekiel. This vision involves complex geometric shapes and fiery creatures and is interpreted by some as a symbolic representation of God's power and majesty.

When I use the term Merkaba, also written Mer-Ka-Ba or Merkabah, I am referring to a geometric energy field surrounding the human body. These spirals of electromagnetic energy exist around and within all forms. It is a star tetrahedron or two interlocked tetrahedrons forming a star shape. The top and bottom tetrahedrons spiral in counter-rotating directions and continually expand and contract the perpetual supply of renewed energy radiation into and out of manifestation.[106] The upper tetrahedron is electrical, and the lower is magnetic.[51]

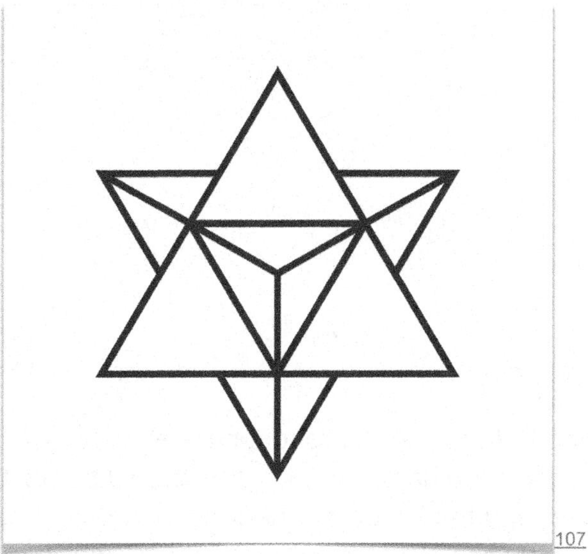
[107]

A two-dimensional star tetrahedron reminds me of the Star of David in Judaism. Breaking the word down, Mer refers to source force movement, Ka refers to source force expression, and Ba refers to vehicle.

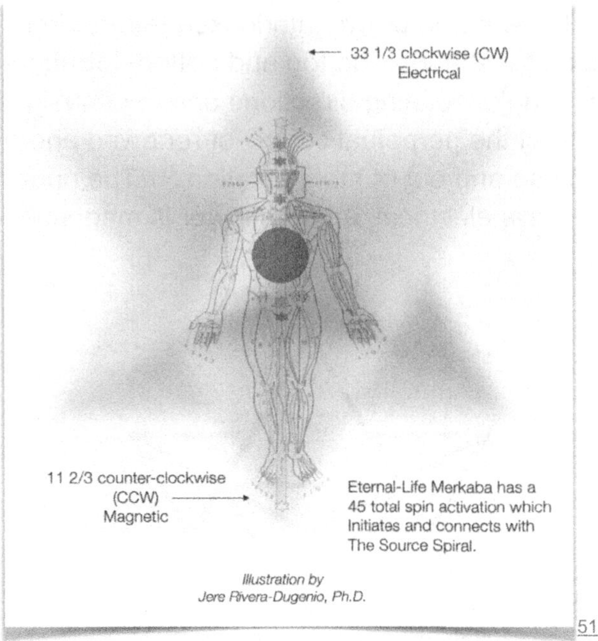

[51]

According to Quantum Morphogenetic Physics, the spin-speed ratio of the upper tetrahedron should be 33 1/3 clockwise, and the lower tetrahedron should be 11 2/3 counterclockwise. This spin ratio totals 45, which is considered an eternal mathematical number. Use caution when studying Merakabas, as people teach that the spin should total 55, which will phase-lock you into your current reality.

PART DD

(dd) **Create coherence with X, Y, and Z planes.**

Refer to Part BB for the word "**coherence**."

The three-dimensional Cartesian coordinate system uses the X, Y, and X planes. Each plane is perpendicular to the other two planes.

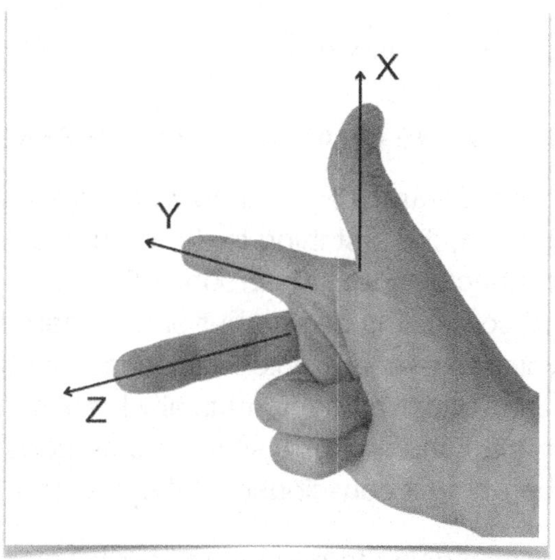

Each of the three planes has rotation around it from two opposite directions. I envision creating coherence in all the elements of the human body and fields in all three planes, including rotation in both directions in those three planes.

There are times in a clearing when specific tissues, organs, or body areas do not have cohesion in one or more of the planes associated with rotation in one way or another. In those cases, restoring coherence allows all the parts to be optimally connected and working in unison.

Chapter 5. When the Clear It Template is Done

Adapting To The Change That Happened

After using the Clear It Template to work on someone besides yourself, the first thing to do when you finish is break all connections to that person. Otherwise, you can have a cord connecting each other or the energy fields between you can overlap, which will cause interference. My friend Dr. Todd Watts automatically breaks the connection after the patient visit so that he does not have to remember to do it consciously at the end of the visit.

When you finish going through the Clear It Template for yourself, it can take 10-15 minutes for your body and energetics to get readjusted to the release and the new energetic status.

I like to do a few things to help facilitate and speed up the adaptation. The first thing I typically do is stand up and walk around. I also like to stretch my arms, back, and legs. I tend to yawn a couple of times while my body resets. I will often use the bathroom and blow my nose.

I find doing breathing techniques with visualization to be helpful. In her book "The Energy Codes," Dr. Sue Morter teaches a methodology called Central Channel Breathing that I think works well. I visualize that I am bringing Earth's energy up through my feet into my body as I breathe in. I focus on moving that energy up through my body to the areas that feel stuck or are off. I visualize that I am picking up that stuck or negative energy. Then I breathe that air out through the top of my head and send it back to the heavens, God, or source.

I will then go in the opposite direction. As I breathe in, I visualize bringing the energies from the heavens, God, or source down through my head and into my body. I move that energy around the areas that still feel stuck or any new areas I feel. Then, on an exhale, I will push that energy out the bottom of my feet back into Earth.

The goal is to shift energy around the body to create coherence and synergy. The focus is always to sense where there is tension or a gathering of energy stuck in the body. As I breathe the energy in, I bring the air I am pulling into the body directly to those areas. Then on the outbreath I send all the energy out of my body..

In Chapter 1 I mentioned that dogs shake off energy to reset them. That can also be an option for us humans as well.

There is a Hawaiian prayer for forgiveness called Ho'oponopono, pronounced HO-oh-Po-no-Po-no, that is excellent to read four times to reset the body energetically. The prayer reads, "I love you. I am sorry. Please forgive me. Thank you."

I found the above things to help me adjust after the Clear It Template. As always, do what feels best for you.

If you decide to study Quantum Morphogenetic Physics, the program offers advanced effective breathing techniques that help to reset the body energetics as well.

CHAPTER 6. WHAT TO DO WHEN STUCK?

THE BREAKTHROUGH

What does it mean to be stuck? Being stuck is a common human feeling that can be interpreted from a few different things. It can arise from a sense of not progressing in life. It can also come in when you feel uncertain about what to do next. Someone can feel stuck when they lose their motivation and do not want to complete what they've been working on. Having an emotional roadblock, like fear, anxiety, or shame, or even feeling limited in the options you have are ways that the feeling stuck manifests.

In the context of this book and teaching the Clear It Template, you may feel stuck if you stop progressing with eliminating symptoms and improving how you feel.

When you feel stuck, consider the fact you are missing something. This could be a past trauma, current stressor, or an issue that is right in front of your face. Remember, when you have symptoms or feel off, your body is trying to communicate with you. The symptoms disappear when you hear the communication and respond accordingly.

I would love to say that the Clear It Template is the end-all and will fix everything in your life. However, it is simply a tool to grow, expand, and build upon. The purpose of writing this book is to share what I've learned in the last few years that have been transformative for me and to provide you with some tools that impact the unseen world.

When I feel stuck, I tend to go to a quiet space and listen

to the thoughts that come in to see if I will get clues as to what I am missing that manifests this feeling. For me, it has usually been to add, change, or tweak something within the Clear It Template. Since the start of figuring all this out, I have had immense inspiration and motivation to finish and publish this. I do not know where that inspiration and motivation comes from, but it is something I have felt I had to do.

It is important to ask if your intentions are aligned with what results you are seeking. You will continue running into a wall if your goal does not align with your true intentions.

As mentioned in this book, many parts of our lives often require healing, to include physical, chemical, mental, emotional, energetic, spiritual, relationships, career, finances, etc.

If you are feeling stuck, it may not be related to something you have missed in the Clear It Template but to something in one of the above categories, such as a relationship you are in or a job you currently have. The more layers you peel back with the Clear It Template, the easier it is to see what needs to be changed, altered, or worked on in your life.

CHAPTER 7. HOW TO GO DEEPER IN YOUR RELEASE

TIMELINE YOUR LIFE

New German Medicine has a theory that conflicts in your life will repeat until you break or heal its cycle. The New German Medicine's first cycle is from birth until you are at an independent age, which could be at 18 or somewhere typically around that. The age at which you gain independence will vary per person, but it's usually between 18 to 22. It is not just when you move out of the house but when you start living on your terms, including buying groceries, doing your laundry, and being responsible for life.

The New German Medicine timeline is created by starting at year zero, when you were born, until that independent age, which was about 20 years old for me. You take time to go through your timeline of all the different conflicts, significant events, and traumas that occurred each year and write them down. When you are done, you'll have each year written down, including zero, one, two, three, four, etc., to your current age. Your first cycle will be from zero to that independent age, which for me was 20. New German Medicine has found that concentric circles will form in the brain from accumulated conflicts. These conflicts will appear on a brain CT (computer tomogram) scan as a set of concentric rings called "Hamer foci" that look like circles from a cross-section of a tree trunk. When you heal those past conflicts, the concentric circles will heal and fill in, which again can be seen on a CT scan.

When you research New German Medicine, Google®

loves to remind you that it is controversial and lacks scientific basis. I have a practitioner friend who has had personal, impactful health changes based on this work.

Regarding filling in your own timeline of events in your life portion, I encourage asking family members and parents about any significant conflicts and events and what they were. According to New German Medicine, if you had a substantial conflict at age three, that would repeat three years into your second cycle and three years into your third cycle until you heal that past conflict. For example, if your independent age was 20, your second cycle is from 20 through 40. That conflict at age three would resurface at age 23 and, if still not healed, would again resurface when you are 43 and continue until you heal the conflict and break the repeating cycle.

I do not know much more about New German Medicine theories and ideas, but I bring this up because I see the value in creating a timeline of significant conflicts, events, and traumas in your life. Document the age as it becomes a great reference to go back, work through, and clear. The more you can reflect and recall what has happened, the easier it is to release it entirely via the Clear It Template.

Some ideas to help jog your memory on impactful conflicts are thinking about every person you have interacted with in this life experience, such as the following: your parents, siblings, grandparents, kids, grandkids, aunts, uncles, cousins, friends, neighbors, classmates, coworkers, bosses, babysitters, doctors, teachers, coaches, etc.

Think back to each age where you lived and what life was like. The more conscious you are of events and traumas that happened, the easier it is to release them.

As you identify past conflicts, use that specific conflict and memory as the “specific challenge” from Part A when reading through the Clear It Template.

If there is a particular area of your body that you tend to favor, protect, unconsciously hold, touch often or have pain in, that is a clue that there is something to release.

To go deeper, consider what your intuitive mind leads you to. Often, when I am quiet, I will get random fleeting thoughts that help to give me clues as to how to go deeper or bring up areas that need attention.

“The intuitive mind is a sacred gift, and the rational mind is a faithful servant. We have created a society that honors the servant and has forgotten the gift.” ~Albert Einstein

CHAPTER 8. SAVE TIME

WHAT DO THE BOLDED WORDS MEAN?

When reading through the Clear It Template, you will notice bolded words at the beginning of a sentence or section.

You can expedite reading through the Clear It Template by only reading the bolded words. These words hold the entire intention of everything not bolded in the Clear It Template.

While reading through just the bolded words will ultimately save time, it is essential to dive deeply into the Clear It Template, including what each word and phrase means. Once you fully understand it, you can feel free to use the shortened version by reciting the bolded words and phrases. The result of grasping every part of the template and its purpose will be an expanded awareness and more impactful results.

Fate favors action!

About the Author

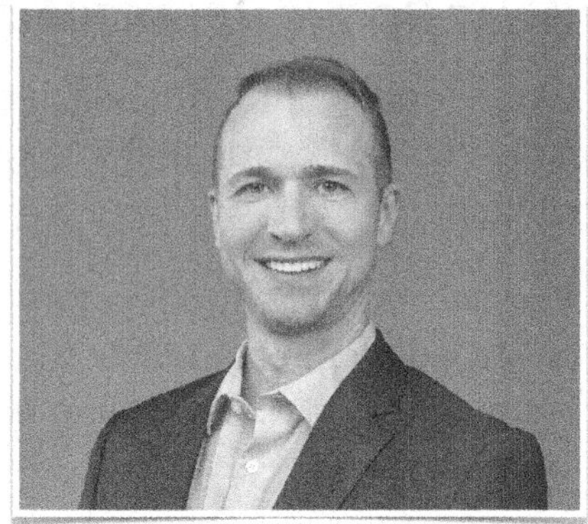

After nearly losing his wife Heather, a doctor herself, to Lyme disease, Dr. Jay Davidson learned through trial and error what was needed to save her life. Once she recovered, he used his discoveries to create healing protocols for CellCore Biosciences. CellCore is a practitioner health supplement company Dr. Davidson co-founded with Dr. Todd Watts. CellCore creates natural solutions for gut, immune, and whole-body health.

Dr. Davidson completed his undergraduate studies at the University of Wisconsin La Crosse and majored in biology with a biomedical concentration and chemistry minor. He received his Doctor of Chiropractic at the Northwestern College of Chiropractic in Minnesota.

As a two-time #1 international best-selling author, Dr. Davidson is admired for his ability to bridge the gap between the scientific health community and the layperson. A veracious learner, he is constantly seeking the most cutting-edge information that will improve his ability to help others on their healing journeys. He believes in being intentionally disruptive by innovating, creating, and leaning into the inner call to change the world.

Can I Ask You For a Favor?

If you find value in this book, I would appreciate you posting a review on Amazon.

I appreciate your support!

REFERENCES

1. Wikipedia contributors. (2023, September 24). *List of religions and spiritual traditions*. Wikipedia. https://en.m.wikipedia.org/wiki/List_of_religions_and_spiritual_traditions
2. Wikipedia contributors. (2024a, January 11). *List of organs of the human body*. Wikipedia. https://en.wikipedia.org/wiki/List_of_organs_of_the_human_body
3. Cowan, P. T. (2023, November 13). *Anatomy, bones*. StatPearls - NCBI Bookshelf. https://www.ncbi.nlm.nih.gov/books/NBK537199/
4. Seladi-Schulman, J., PhD. (2020, February 4). *How many muscles are in the human body?* Healthline. https://www.healthline.com/health/how-many-muscles-are-in-the-human-body
5. Sender, R., Fuchs, S., & Milo, R. (2016). Revised Estimates for the Number of Human and Bacteria Cells in the Body. *PLoS biology, 14*(8), e1002533. https://doi.org/10.1371/journal.pbio.1002533
6. Lee, E. (2019, May 26). We're only about 43% human, study shows. *Voice of America*. https://www.voanews.com/a/research-estimates-we-are-only-about-43-percent-human/4932876.html
7. Alberts, B. (2002). *The chemical components of a cell*. Molecular Biology of the Cell - NCBI Bookshelf. https://www.ncbi.nlm.nih.gov/books/NBK26883/
8. Cole, L. A., & Kramer, P. R. (2016). Macronutrients. In *Elsevier eBooks* (pp. 157–164). https://doi.org/10.1016/b978-0-12-803699-0.00005-0
9. Valenzuela, B. R., & Valenzuela, B. (2013). Overview about lipid structure. In *InTech eBooks*. https://doi.org/10.5772/52306
10. Sparkman, O. D., Penton, Z. E., & Kitson, F. G. (2011). Amino acids. *In Elsevier eBooks* (pp. 265–

271). https://doi.org/10.1016/b978-0-12-373628-4.00012-5

11. *Nucleotide*. (n.d.). Genome.gov. https://www.genome.gov/genetics-glossary/Nucleotide
12. Wikipedia contributors. (2024b, January 30). *Nucleotide*. Wikipedia. https://en.wikipedia.org/wiki/Nucleotide
13. Schirber, M. (2009, April 16). The chemistry of life: The human body. *livescience.com*. https://www.livescience.com/3505-chemistry-life-human-body.html
14. Randjelovic, E. (2018, March 3). *Bohr model of Oxygen Atom with proton, neutron and electron. Science*. . . iStock. https://www.istockphoto.com/photo/bohr-model-of-oxygen-atom-with-proton-neutron-and-electron-gm926457798-254203266
15. Randjelovic, E. (2018a, March 3). *Bohr model of Hydrogen Atom with proton and electron. Science and*. . . iStock. https://www.istockphoto.com/photo/bohr-model-of-hydrogen-atom-with-proton-and-electron-gm926457788-254203258
16. Sarkar, N. (2021, December 25). *Isotopes of Carbon. Atomic Structure of Carbon-12, Carbon-13 and*. . . iStock. https://www.istockphoto.com/vector/isotopes-of-carbon-3d-vector-illustration-gm1360655261-433592347
17. Google® search results from (2023, November 27) https://homework.study.com/explanation/what-percentage-of-the-atom-is-empty-space.html
18. ThunderboltsProject. (2023, January 15). *Michael Armstrong: Aether is Squidgy | Thunderbolts* [Video]. YouTube. https://www.youtube.com/watch?v=vJQPoBFQwbw
19. Soedarto, G. (2023, February 21). Albert Einstein began by rejecting the ether theory. . .. .

Medium. https://medium.com/@GatotSoedarto/albert-einstein-began-by-rejecting-the-ether-theory-2e0d8ff8a812

20. Rivera-Dugenio, J., PhD. (2019, January). The evolution of consciousness to matter. *International Journal of Scientific & Engineering Research* Volume 10, Issue 1, P594-600 ISSN 2229-5518 https://www.ijser.org/researchpaper/The-Evolution-of-Consciousness-to-Matter.pdf
21. WaySide. (2021, July 16). The Rockefellers, The Flexner Report, The AMA, And Their Effect On Alternative Nutritional (botanical). *TRUTH IN PLAIN SIGHT*. https://truthinplainsight.com/the-rockefellers-the-flexner-report-the-ama-and-their-effect-on-alternative-nutritional-botanical-medicine/
22. Wright-Mendoza, J. (2019). The 1910 report that disadvantaged minority doctors. *JSTOR Daily*. https://daily.jstor.org/the-1910-report-that-unintentionally-disadvantaged-minority-doctors/
23. Duffy, T. P. (2011, September 1). *The Flexner Report — 100 years later*. PubMed Central (PMC). https://www.ncbi.nlm.nih.gov/pmc/articles/PMC3178858/
24. K. Meyl (2011b) *DNA—reading and writing by scalar waves*. 2nd World DNA Day—China, 2011, Track 2.7, conf. proc., p.101
25. Rivera-Dugenio, J., PhD. (2019, April). The Language of Our DNA – Scalar Energy. *International Journal of Scientific & Engineering Research* Volume 10, Issue 4, P212-218 ISSN 2229-5518 https://www.ijser.org/researchpaper/The-Language-of-Our-DNA-Scalar-Energy.pdf
26. Wikipedia contributors. (2024b, January 16). *Quantum entanglement*. Wikipedia. https://en.wikipedia.org/wiki/Quantum_entanglement

27. *The Nobel Prize in Physics 2022*. (n.d.). NobelPrize.org. https://www.nobelprize.org/prizes/physics/2022/press-release/
28. Wikipedia contributors. (2024f, February 15). *List of religions and spiritual traditions*. Wikipedia. https://en.m.wikipedia.org/wiki/List_of_religions_and_spiritual_traditions
29. Lu, M. (2022, June 20). *Visualizing the world's most popular religions*. Visual Capitalist. https://www.visualcapitalist.com/cp/visualizing-religions-worldwide/
30. Wikipedia contributors. (2024d, February 9). *Christian denomination*. Wikipedia. https://en.wikipedia.org/wiki/Christian_denomination
31. Snibbe, K., & Gqlshare. (2023, April 8). You might be surprised at how many Christian denominations there are in the world. *Orange County Register*. https://www.ocregister.com/2023/04/07/you-might-be-surprised-at-how-many-christian-denominations-there-are-in-the-world/
32. transmute. (2024). In *Merriam-Webster Dictionary*. https://www.merriam-webster.com/dictionary/transmute
33. transmutation. (n.d.). In *Merriam-Webster Dictionary*. https://www.merriam-webster.com/dictionary/transmutation
34. Wikipedia contributors. (2023, December 28). *Three corpses*. Wikipedia. https://en.wikipedia.org/wiki/Three_Corpses
35. Wikipedia contributors. (2024h, February 16). *Succubus*. Wikipedia. https://en.wikipedia.org/wiki/Succubus
36. Wikipedia contributors. (2024c, January 19). *Tenacious D (album)*. Wikipedia. https://en.wikipedia.org/wiki/Tenacious_D_(album)

37. *Amazon.in.* (n.d.). https://www.amazon.in/Tenacious-D-12th-Anniversary-Vinyl/dp/B00AYJBS5I
38. Bob Dylan gives rare interview. (2016, October 13). *CBS News.* https://www.cbsnews.com/news/60-minutes-bob-dylan-rare-interview-2004/
39. Start To Continue. (2021, September 21). *Bob Dylan FULL 60 Minutes Ed Bradley 2004 Interview (upscaled to HD)* [Video]. YouTube. https://youtube.com/watch?v=hOas0d-fFK8&si=EnSlkaIECMiOmarE&t=842
40. *Beyoncé on her alter ego, Sasha Fierce*. (n.d.). [Video]. Oprah.com. https://www.oprah.com/own-oprahshow/beyonc-on-her-alter-ego-sasha-fierce
41. OWN. (2019, August 17). *Beyoncé on her alter ego, Sasha Fierce | The Oprah Winfrey Show | Oprah Winfrey Network* [Video]. YouTube. https://www.youtube.com/watch?v=4AA5G8vCl9w
42. *What is Mind Field Repatterning™ | Awakening Hearts and Minds*. (n.d.). Mysite. https://www.awakeningheartsandminds.com/what-is-mind-field-repatterning-tm
43. *Raymon Grace*. (n.d.). Raymon Grace. https://www.raymongrace.us/#/
44. Analysis and assessment of Gateway Process. (n.d.). https://www.cia.gov/readingroom/docs/CIA-RDP96-00788R001700210016-5.pdf
45. *What is the simulation hypothesis? Why some think life is a simulated reality*. (2018, October 3). NBC News. https://www.nbcnews.com/mach/science/what-simulation-hypothesis-why-some-think-life-simulated-reality-ncna913926
46. Image from https://www.reddit.com/media?url=https%3A%2F%2Fi.redd.it%2F32auojf9fqr91.jpg
47. *Are you living in a simulation?* (n.d.). https://simulation-argument.com/simulation

48. Recode. (2016, June 2). *Is life a video game? | Elon Musk | Code Conference 2016* [Video]. YouTube. https://www.youtube.com/watch?v=2KK_kzrJPS8
49. Bsajk. (2023, March 31). *20230331 – WHY WOO*. Clif High Videos. https://clifhighvideos.com/20230331a/
50. *WHY Woo*. (n.d.). BitChute. https://www.bitchute.com/video/OF8GfTaw7mcD/
51. Rivera-Dugenio, J., PhD. *Level-One, Level-Two, and Level-Three lecture notes*. BioRegenesis Academy. https://www.bioregenesisacademy.org/
52. Dolega, M. E., Monnier, S., Brunel, B., Joanny, J., Recho, P., & Cappello, G. (2021). Extracellular matrix in multicellular aggregates acts as a pressure sensor controlling cell proliferation and motility. *eLife*, 10. https://doi.org/10.7554/elife.63258
53. Rau, T. (2011). *Biological medicine - the future of natural healing*.
54. Steen B. (1997). Body water in the elderly--a review. *The journal of nutrition, health & aging*, *1*(3), 142–145. https://pubmed.ncbi.nlm.nih.gov/10995081/
55. Melouane, A., Yoshioka, M., & St-Amand, J. (2020). Extracellular matrix/mitochondria pathway: A novel potential target for sarcopenia. *Mitochondrion, 50*, 63–70. https://doi.org/10.1016/j.mito.2019.10.007
56. Urra, F. A., Fuentes-Retamal, S., Palominos, C., Rodríguez-Lucart, Y. A., López-Torres, C., & Araya-Maturana, R. (2021). Extracellular matrix signals as drivers of mitochondrial bioenergetics and metabolic plasticity of cancer cells during metastasis. *Frontiers in Cell and Developmental Biology, 9*. https://doi.org/10.3389/fcell.2021.751301
57. Lesondak, D., & Akey, A. M. (2020). *Fascia, function, and medical applications*.

58. Montagnier, L., Del Giudice, E., Aïssa, J., Lavallée, C., Motschwiller, S., Capolupo, A., Polcari, A., Romano, P., Tedeschi, A., & Vitiello, G. (2015). Transduction of DNA information through water and electromagnetic waves. *Electromagnetic Biology and Medicine, 34*(2), 106–112. https://doi.org/10.3109/15368378.2015.1036072
59. Gałęcki, R., & Sokół, R. (2019). A parasitological evaluation of edible insects and their role in the transmission of parasitic diseases to humans and animals. *PLOS ONE, 14*(7), e0219303. https://doi.org/10.1371/journal.pone.0219303
60. BOE.es - Sumario del día 17/04/2020. (2020, April 17). https://www.boe.es/boe/dias/2020/04/17/
61. The full document was accessed (2022, June 14) https://www.boe.es/boe/dias/2020/04/17/pdfs/BOE-A-2020-4492.pdf
62. Screenshot from Google® search result from "biocide" (2022, June 14)
63. Earth, D. O. (1997). Toxicologic assessment of the army's zinc cadmium sulfide dispersion tests. In *National Academies Press eBooks*. https://doi.org/10.17226/5739
64. Wikipedia contributors. (2023a, December 18). *Operation Sea-Spray*. Wikipedia. https://en.wikipedia.org/wiki/Operation_Sea-Spray
65. *Lab tests*. (2022, February 8). Geoengineering Watch. https://www.geoengineeringwatch.org/lab-tests-2/
66. *170 million in U.S. drink radioactive tap water*. (2018, January 11). Environmental Working Group. https://www.ewg.org/research/170-million-us-drink-radioactive-tap-water
67. Sevostianova, E., Lindemann, W. C., Ulery, A., & Remmenga, M. D. (2010). Plant Uptake of Depleted Uranium from Manure-Amended and Citrate Treated Soil. *International Journal of Phytoremediation, 12*(6), 550–561. https://doi.org/10.1080/15226510903353153

68. *How to access the TSCA inventory | US EPA.* (2023, August 16). US EPA. https://www.epa.gov/tsca-inventory/how-access-tsca-inventory
69. *The Agent Orange in Vietnam program - The Aspen Institute*. (2023, October 25). The Aspen Institute. https://www.aspeninstitute.org/programs/agent-orange-in-vietnam-program/
70. *Dioxin contamination in Viet Nam: Emissions from industries and levels in the environment.* (n.d.). Viet Nam. https://vietnam.un.org/en/13566-dioxin-contamination-viet-nam-emissions-industries-and-levels-environment
71. Schecter, A., Pavúk, M., Malisch, R., & Ryan, J. (2003). Are Vietnamese Food Exports Contaminated with Dioxin from Agent Orange? *Journal of Toxicology and Environmental Health, Part A: Current Issues, 66*(15–16), 1391–1404. https://doi.org/10.1080/15287390306416
72. Luo, Y., Gibson, C. T., Chuah, C., Tang, Y., Naidu, R., & Fang, C. (2022). Raman imaging for the identification of Teflon microplastics and nanoplastics released from non-stick cookware. *Science of the Total Environment, 851*, 158293. https://doi.org/10.1016/j.scitotenv.2022.158293
73. Emily Main for Rodalenews.com. (2022, April 5). Your bottled water has 24,500 chemicals. *Prevention*. https://www.prevention.com/food-nutrition/healthy-eating/a20459644/your-bottled-water-has-24-500-chemicals/
74. Landa, J. (2015, October 27). More than 24,500 chemicals found in bottled water. *Fox News*. https://www.foxnews.com/health/more-than-24500-chemicals-found-in-bottled-water
75. Healing, D. (2024, January 3). *Discover Energy Healing with The Emotion Code® | Discover Healing*. Discover Healing. https://discoverhealing.com/

76. Bordoni, B. (2023, July 17). *Anatomy, fascia.* StatPearls - NCBI Bookshelf. https://www.ncbi.nlm.nih.gov/books/NBK493232/
77. Felitti, V. J., Anda, R. F., Nordenberg, D., Williamson, D. F., Spitz, A. M., Edwards, V. J., Koss, M. P., & Marks, J. S. (1998). Relationship of childhood abuse and household dysfunction to many of the leading causes of death in adults. *American Journal of Preventive Medicine, 14*(4), 245–258. https://doi.org/10.1016/s0749-3797(98)00017-8
78. Centers for Disease Control and Prevention. (2021, April 6). *About the CDC-Kaiser Ace Study | Violence prevention | injury Center* | CDC. Centers for Disease Control and Prevention. https://www.cdc.gov/violenceprevention/aces/about.html
79. empathy. (2024). In *Merriam-Webster Dictionary.* https://www.merriam-webster.com/dictionary/empathy
80. Bordoni, B., Marelli, F., Bruno, M., & Sacconi, B. (2018). Emission of biophotons and adjustable sounds by the fascial system: review and reflections for manual therapy. *Journal of Evidence-Based Integrative Medicine, 23,* 2515690X1775075. https://doi.org/10.1177/2515690x17750750
81. Pajić-Lijaković, I., Milivojević, M., & Clark, A. G. (2022). Collective cell migration on Collagen-I networks: The impact of matrix viscoelasticity. *Frontiers in Cell and Developmental Biology, 10.* https://doi.org/10.3389/fcell.2022.901026
82. Samsel, A., & Seneff, S. (2016). Glyphosate pathways to modern diseases V: Amino acid analogue of glycine in diverse proteins. *Journal of Biological Physics and Chemistry, 16*(1), 9–46. https://doi.org/10.4024/03sa16a.jbpc.16.01
83. Costas-Ferreira, C., Durán, R., & Faro, L. (2022). Toxic effects of glyphosate on the nervous system:

a systematic review. *International Journal of Molecular Sciences, 23*(9), 4605. https://doi.org/10.3390/ijms23094605

84. Liptan, G. (2010). Fascia: A missing link in our understanding of the pathology of fibromyalgia. *Journal of Bodywork and Movement Therapies, 14*(1), 3–12. https://doi.org/10.1016/j.jbmt.2009.08.003
85. PeterHermesFurian. (2014, April 4). *Illustration of a meditating woman in yoga position with the seven...* iStock. https://www.istockphoto.com/vector/chakras-woman-with-description-gm482901779-37500228
86. Delbert, C. (2022, February 21). Earth pulsates every 26 seconds. no one knows why. *Popular Mechanics*. https://www.popularmechanics.com/science/environment/a34531984/earth-pulsates-every-26-seconds/
87. Elhalel, G., Price, C., Fixler, D., & Shainberg, A. (2019). Cardioprotection from stress conditions by weak magnetic fields in the Schumann Resonance band. *Scientific Reports, 9*(1). https://doi.org/10.1038/s41598-018-36341-z
88. *Schumann Resonance.* (n.d.). MRMBB333. https://www.mrmbb333.com/schumann-resonance.html
89. Fdez-Arróyabe, P., Fornieles-Callejón, J., Santurtún, A., Szangolies, L., & Donner, R. V. (2020). Schumann resonance and cardiovascular hospital admission in the area of Granada, Spain: An event coincidence analysis approach. *Science of the Total Environment, 705*, 135813. https://doi.org/10.1016/j.scitotenv.2019.135813
90. Alabdulgader, A., McCraty, R., Atkinson, M., Dobyns, Y., Vainoras, A., Ragulskis, M., & Štolc, V. (2018). Long-Term study of heart rate variability responses to changes in the solar and geomagnetic

environment. *Scientific Reports, 8*(1). https://doi.org/10.1038/s41598-018-20932-x

91. Direnfeld, L. (1983). The Genesis of the EEG and its Relation to Electromagnetic Radiation. *Journal of Bioelectricity, 2*(2–3), 111–121. https://doi.org/10.3109/15368378309009845
92. Tracy, S. M., Vieira, C. L., Garshick, E., Wang, V. A., Alahmad, B., Eid, R., Schwartz, J., Schiff, J. E., Vokonas, P., & Koutrakis, P. (2022). Associations between solar and geomagnetic activity and peripheral white blood cells in the Normative Aging Study. *Environmental Research, 204*, 112066. https://doi.org/10.1016/j.envres.2021.112066
93. Tang, J. Y., Yeh, T. W., Huang, Y., Wang, M. H., & Jang, L. S. (2019). Effects of extremely low-frequency electromagnetic fields on B16F10 cancer cells. *Electromagnetic Biology and Medicine, 38*(2), 149–157. https://doi.org/10.1080/15368378.2019.1591438
94. Zimecki M. (2006). The lunar cycle: effects on human and animal behavior and physiology. *Postepy higieny i medycyny doswiadczalnej (Online)*, *60*, 1–7. https://pubmed.ncbi.nlm.nih.gov/16407788/
95. Blank, M., & Goodman, R. (2011). DNA is a fractal antenna in electromagnetic fields. *International Journal of Radiation Biology, 87*(4), 409–415. https://doi.org/10.3109/09553002.2011.538130
96. Armour J. A. (2007). The little brain on the heart. *Cleveland Clinic journal of medicine*, *74 Suppl 1*, S48–S51. https://doi.org/10.3949/ccjm.74.suppl_1.s48
97. Rivera-Dugenio, J., PhD. (2020, January). 12-Strand DNA Morphogenetic Engineering Via Holofractal Morphogenetic Reprogramming of Genetic Information. *International Journal of Scientific & Engineering Research* Volume 11, Issue 1, P950-963 ISSN 2229-5518 https://www.ijser.org/researchpaper/12-Strand-

DNA-Morphogenetic-Engineering-Via-Holofractal-Morphogenetic-Reprogramming-of-Genetic-Information.pdf

98. Markel, H. (2021). *The secret of life: Rosalind Franklin, James Watson, Francis Crick, and the Discovery of DNA's Double Helix*. National Geographic Books.
99. Biffi, G., Tannahill, D., McCafferty, J., & Balasubramanian, S. (2013). Quantitative visualization of DNA G-quadruplex structures in human cells. *Nature Chemistry, 5*(3), 182–186. https://doi.org/10.1038/nchem.1548
100. *Mutation*. (n.d.). Genome.gov. https://www.genome.gov/genetics-glossary/Mutation
101. Sheldrake, R. (2009). *Morphic resonance: The Nature of Formative Causation*. Inner Traditions / Bear & Co.
102. Sheldrake, R. (n.d.). *A new science of life / morphic resonance*. Rupert Sheldrake – Author and Biologist. https://www.sheldrake.org/books-by-rupert-sheldrake/a-new-science-of-life-morphic-resonance
103. Kjellqvist, A., Palmquist, E., & Nordin, S. (2016). Psychological symptoms and health-related quality of life in idiopathic environmental intolerance attributed to electromagnetic fields. *Journal of psychosomatic research, 84*, 8–12. https://doi.org/10.1016/j.jpsychores.2016.03.006
104. Zimmerman, F. J., Von Saint André-Von Arnim, A., & McLaughlin, J. L. (2011). Cellular respiration. In *Elsevier eBooks* (pp. 1058–1072). https://doi.org/10.1016/b978-0-323-07307-3.10074-6
105. Davis, A. R., & Rawls, W. C. (1974). Magnetism and its effects on the living system. Hicksville, N.Y. : Exposition Press, 1974, 1976 printing.

106. *Merkaba - the vehicle of light*. (2023, February 11). Chintamania. https://www.chintamania.com/single-post/merkaba-the-vehicle-of-light

107. Vector, T. (2022, November 6). *3D object that is made out of two triangles facing opposite. . .* iStock. https://www.istockphoto.com/vector/merkaba-symbol-sacred-geometry-shape-star-tetrahedron-gm1438850205-479251580

Made in United States
Orlando, FL
04 May 2024

46500315R00085